KETO BREAD COOKBOOK

80 EASY AND EXCITING LOW CARB KETO BREAD BAKING RECIPES FOR FAST WEIGHT LOSS

NICOLE JAMES

Legal & Disclaimer

The information contained in this book and its contents is not designed to replace or take the place of any form of medical or professional advice; and is not meant to replace the need for independent medical, financial, legal or other professional advice or services, as may be required. The content and information in this book has been provided for educational and entertainment purposes only.

The content and information contained in this book has been compiled from sources deemed reliable, and it is accurate to the best of the Author's knowledge, information and belief. However, the Author cannot guarantee its accuracy and validity and cannot be held liable for any errors and/or omissions. Further, changes are periodically made to this book as and when needed. Where appropriate and/or necessary, you must consult a professional (including but not limited to your doctor, attorney, financial advisor or such other professional advisor) before using any of the suggested remedies, techniques, or information in this book.

Upon using the contents and information contained in this book, you agree to hold harmless the Author from and against any damages, costs, and expenses, including any legal fees potentially resulting from the application of any of the information provided by this book. This disclaimer applies to any loss, damages or injury caused by the use and application, whether directly or indirectly, of any advice or information presented, whether for breach of contract, tort, negligence, personal injury, criminal intent, or under any other cause of action.

You agree to accept all risks of using the information presented inside this book.

You agree that by continuing to read this book, where appropriate and/or necessary, you shall consult a professional (including but not limited to your doctor, attorney, or financial advisor or such other advisor as needed) before using any of the suggested remedies, techniques, or information in this book.

TABLE OF CONTENTS

TABLE OF CONTENTS 3

Free Bonus 7

Guide To Low Carb Flours And Sweeteners To Use In Baking 8

Almond Flour 11

Whey or Egg White Protein Powder 12

Psyllium Husk Powder and Psyllium Husks Whole.................12

Organic Coconut Flour...13

Organic Sesame Flour...13

Ground Flaxseed..13

Stevia..14

Allulose..14

Erythritol..14

Basic Breads 15

1. Keto Dinner Rolls 16

2. Keto Sandwich Bread 17

3. Keto Cinnamon Rolls 18

4. Keto Bread Sticks 20

5. Keto Banana Loaf 21

6. Keto English Muffins..23

7. Keto Biscuits 24

8. Keto Garlic Bread...25

9. Keto Aurora Toast..26

10. Keto Zucchini Bread..28

11. Keto Cloud Bread 29

12. Keto Bagels 30

13. Keto Pull-Apart Rolls 31

14. Keto Cauliflower Bread 32

15. Keto Cheese Bread 33

16. Keto Mug Bread 34

17. Keto Blender Buns 35

18. Keto Ciabatta 36

19. Keto Burger Buns 37

20. Keto Pizza Crust 38

Flatbreads **39**

1. Coco-Cilantro Flatbread 40

2. Almond Curry Naan 41

3. Chili and Cheese Tortillas 42

4. Garlic-Parmesan Chapati 43

5. Avocado Flatbread 44

6. Sun-Dried Tomato and Parsley Pitas 45

7. Onion Roti 46

8. Butter Parsley Flatbread 47

9. Spiced Soft Tacos 48

10. Spinach and Cheese Tortillas 49

Muffins & Cupcakes **50**

1. Blueberry and Cream Cheese Muffins 51

2. Ham and Parmesan Muffins 52

3. Cheddar Jalapeno Muffins 53

4. Chocolate Zucchini Muffins 54

5. Broccoli and Cheese Muffins 55

6. Carrot Cardamom Muffins 56

7. Squash and Cinnamon Muffins 57

8. Keto Red Velvet Muffins 58

9. Coffee Butter Muffins 59

10. Choco Peanut Butter Muffins 60

11. Lemon Butter Cupcakes 61

12. Three-Cheese Cupcakes 62

13. Cinnamon Sugar Cupcakes 63

14. Strawberry Cream Cheese Cupcakes 64

15. Coco-Blueberry Cupcakes 65

16. Choco-Hazelnut Cupcakes 66

17. Cheddar and Spinach Cupcakes 67

18. Mango-Cayenne Cupcakes 68

19. Lime and Vanilla Cupcakes 69

20. Chia Chocolate Cupcakes 70

Cookies **71**

1. Low-Carb Chocolate Chip Cookies 72

2. Keto Peanut Butter Cookies 73

3. Matcha Coconut Cookies 74

4. Apricot and Cream Cheese Cookies 75

5. Almond Butter Cookies 76

6. Choco Hazelnut Butter Cookies 77

7. Banana Walnut Cookies 78

8. Cinnamon Butter Cookies 79

9. Keto Ginger Cookies 80

10. Low-Carb Butter Pecan Cookies 81

Pancakes **82**

1. Almond Banana Pancakes 83

2. Jalapeno and Cream Cheese Pancakes 84

3. Coconut Chia Pancakes 85

4. Keto Blueberry Pancakes *86*

5. Spiced Pumpkin Pancakes *87*

6. Low-Carb Red Velvet Pancakes *88*

7. Citrus and Ricotta Pancakes *89*

8. Keto Bacon and Cheese Pancakes *90*

9. Keto Avocado Pancakes *91*

10. Purple Yam Pancakes *92*

No-Bake ***93***

1. No-Bake Carrot Cake *94*

2. No-Bake Keto Brownies *95*

3. No-Bake Keto Cheesecake *96*

4. No-Bake Peanut Butter Cookies *97*

5. No-Bake Coconut Bars *98*

6. No-Bake Keto Mousse Cake *99*

7. No-Bake Pumpkin Pie *100*

8. No-Bake Tiramisu Cups *101*

9. No-Bake Choco-Chip Blondies *102*

10. No-Bake Banana Bread *103*

Conclusion ***104***

Free Bonus ***105***

Free Bonus

Thank you for purchasing this cookbook! As a token of my appreciation, I want to give one of my favorite cookbooks for free – "Keto Smoothies: Delicious High-Fat Smoothies To Lose Weight, Boost Energy and Brain Power"

It shows you how to make delicious keto smoothies without ever going out of ketosis. I make these smoothies every day!

To download it, go to HTTPS://WWW.NJKETO.COM/SMOOTHIES and sign up.

After signing up download link will be delivered straight to your mailbox.

By signing up you also agree to receive occasional goodness packed emails from me.

Thank you for reading and enjoying my keto cookbooks!

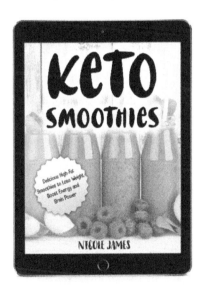

VISIT

HTTPS://WWW.NJKETO.COM/SMOOTHIES

FOR A FREE DOWNLOAD!

Guide To Low Carb Flours And Sweeteners To Use In Baking

Choosing a diet that's right for you can be excessively difficult, especially when you love so many foods that are suddenly placed on the "off limits" list.

But, there is a struggle there as you fight to find the diet that is right for you, that will give you the results that you are craving, and that will fit into the lifestyle you currently live. Because, though you know you should probably make some changes here and there, and if you are going to achieve the results you hope for, it's going to require you do give up on some of the things you love.

This all seems really easy, and even easier when you see the results starting to show. Suddenly, the numbers on the scale begin to drop, your clothes are fitting you differently, and you feel better than ever. Perhaps you are even sleeping better and getting sick less often.

Whatever your goals are, you can see that with the little changes you have made, you are getting closer to achieving those goals.

But then reality sets in.

Our diets...both as a society and branching out into the global world, revolves strongly around bread and bread products in one way or another.

Of course when you think about the foods you are giving up for a new diet, bread is rarely on the list right away.

There are a lot of foods you suddenly can't have, no matter how badly you want them. Though on the outset of the diet you didn't think you were going to miss certain foods, now that you can't have them anymore, it seems like the hardest thing in the world.

You see these foods everywhere, and suddenly the list of foods you now consider staples feel tasteless and bland. You need to get hold of some of that food from your past but you don't sacrifice the changes you have already made in order to do it.

You know bread is on this list. You loved bread, and though you thought it was going to be simple to give it up, it wasn't long before you realized that bread is a large enough staple in your day, you now can't imagine a life without it, and you would do anything to be able to enjoy it again.

From bread on the side of dinner to bread being the main course, suddenly, bread is all you can think about and the only thing that sounds good.

But bread is loaded with carbs and gluten, things you are supposed to be avoiding. This puts you at a crossroad. You know what you want, but you are also dedicated to your diet, and you don't want to stress about cheating on that.

But you are dying for that loaf of bread, and it doesn't seem as though there is any way you are going to get it.

Don't misunderstand me, I am aware that many people have tried their hand at making gluten-free bread, and that there are many, many options on the market today.

Perhaps you have tried your hand at grain free bread making before. As you are aware, there are many people who feel the same way about this as you do, and they are going to do whatever they can to remedy the situation. But, when it comes to baking bread the untraditional way, you are bound to run into your fair share of issues.

Many different grain free breads are dry and crumbly, and they tend to have a flat flavor. Many also call for foods that aren't exactly considered to be real food, meaning you have to compromise in your diet plan in another way if you want the bread.

The secret to the success of your grain free bread lies in both the quality of the ingredients you use, as well as the type of ingredients you use.

In other words, don't be afraid to use real, and experiment with what works for you.

As you will see, the recipes in this book rely heavily on coconut flour. Coconut flour is an incredible option if you want something that is light and easy to work with, don't overpower the bread with a lot of its own flavor, and something you can find easily.

Yes, it's true that many people have complained that their coconut flour tends to make the bread dry, but this isn't an issue with the flour itself, but rather, how the flour is being used. When it comes to using the flour, you have to compensate with other ingredients, in this case, eggs.

Eggs are an excellent way to bring in moisture and buoyancy to your breads without weighing it down with carbs, sweeteners, or anything that goes against what you want to do for yourself.

As you experiment with the recipes in this book, you are going to notice that eggs and coconut flour are present in most, and that the amount of eggs you use is going to be directly affected by the amount of coconut flour in the recipe.

However, even when it comes to such things as coconut flour, coconut oil, and coconut milk, you do have freedom. Choose another kind of flour if you like as highlighted in the next section of the chapter, or try blending flours or using different kinds of oils.

Bear in mind the changes you make are going to affect the flavor of the bread, but for many, the different results add variety and gives them more options with their grain free lifestyle.

All in all, there is going to be a level of trial and error with any recipe you try, especially when you are working with food that has been traditionally prepared a certain way for centuries, but things are constantly growing and changing, and your bread is no exception.

Indulge in all these recipes, and have fun modifying them and turning them into your own. You know you have missed bread, and now is your chance to bring it back into your life not only occasionally, but as often as you want.

****

Before you start baking, you will need some baking essentials to make sure you stick to the keto diet. Some of the products you will need include:

Almond Flour

This is considered one of the best baking alternatives to normal all-purpose flour. Almond flour is grain-free/gluten-free and low carb making it a staple requirement for anyone who is on the keto diet. You can use almond flour to cook all sorts of goodies from breads and cakes to cookies.

You may decide to make the almond flour at the comfort of your home, as all you need is to grind some almonds—for example, in a blender, coffee mill, or spice grinder.

However, you should follow some rules:

- Use only dried or cool almonds.
- Grind a small quantity of almonds at a time.
- Don't grind a portion for over thirty seconds.
- Slightly shake the blender or grinder as you go.

Pour boiling water over the washed nuts several times; peel; simmer; and grind them in a blender, coffee mill or spice grinder. Be careful not to over grind, as from a certain point the almonds will excrete oil, turning your flour into nut-butter. Sift the powder produced at the previous steps and regrind any larger particles.

Such flour is very hygroscopic, which means that it can absorb and retain moisture. Therefore, the almond bakery is less likely to stale and will stay fresh for a longer time.

Almonds are rich in vitamins B, E, and A, as well as in potassium, calcium, iodine, phosphorus, iron, and useful Omega-3 fatty acids. And, they don't lose these useful properties after heating. Almond flour inherits all the health benefits of the nuts and is often used for debilitated patients, people with allergies, and athletes. Some of the most welcomed qualities of almond flour include its ability to reduce/soothe pain, stop seizures, and raise hemoglobin levels; but it's most praised for strengthening heart and blood vessels. However, be careful of nut allergies so as not to harm your health!

It is said that you can never add too many nuts, and almond flour really can contribute to the taste and nutritional value of almost any meal. It's sweet and somewhat milky flavor will make any recipe more festive and distinct, and goes great in any kind of dough, nut-cream, or sweets.

Whey or Egg White Protein Powder

The need for protein powder in baking is simple; it has the same binding effect as gluten, which is not present in low carb recipes. These powders are also great in making keto smoothies.

Psyllium Husk Powder and Psyllium Husks Whole

Psyllium husk powder is an essential product when it comes to baking low carb bread, pies and cakes. It is majorly pure fiber and gives baked foods that bread like texture making it a must-have when it comes to making bread. This product can make low carb breads look exactly like normal white bread but without the excess carbs. When you use it, just make sure you add enough water and eggs and other liquid ingredients because it absorbs a lot of water.

On the other hand, Psyllium husks whole is great for baking low carb tortillas. It will make your tortillas easy to roll out and more elastic.

Organic Coconut Flour

Another gluten-free/grain-free option for baking is coconut flour. This flour contains heat stable fats that make it great for baking. However, you will need to use more liquid ingredients because of its high absorption properties.

Organic Sesame Flour

Flour made from sesame seeds is another awesome option to regular all-purpose flour. It is tasty, makes the perfect keto breads and it has high absorption properties just like coconut flour. Always buy organic sesame flour and use it with Psyllium powder to make your bread fluffy and light.

Ground Flaxseed

In addition to almond and sesame flour, flaxseed flour is another great option that can be used in baking. It has high fiber content and when mixed with water it can be used in place of an egg. Its earthy taste makes it just perfect for making keto friendly breads. You can buy readymade flaxseed flour such as Spectrum Essential Ground Flaxseed or just get whole flaxseeds and grind them, whichever works for you.

While some people believe, our ancestors did not take dairy, most people still think that dairy is a great source of calcium; hence, this book has assumed that you can take dairy in small amounts.

Stevia

This herb is also known as the sugar leaf. It lowers blood pressure, has an anti-inflammatory effect, and can be used by diabetics.

Allulose

Made of natural monosaccharides, this is the most sugar-like sweetener in the market.

Erythritol

This is a substance contained in fruit, vegetables, and sweet corn. It's low in calories and doesn't affect the blood sugar level.

Basic Breads

1. Keto Dinner Rolls

||||||||||||||||||||||||||||||||||||||||||||||||||||||

Looking for a low-carb companion for your favorite dinner stew? Look no further with this awesome recipe.

DETAILS:

- Preparation Time: 10 minutes
- Cooking Time: 12 min
- Serves: 6

NUTRITIONAL VALUES:

- Kcal per serve: 203
- Fat: 17 g. (72%)
- Protein: 9 g. (19%)
- Carbs: 5 g. (9%)

INGREDIENTS:

- 1 cup Almond Flour
- ¼ cup Psyllium Husk Powder
- 1 tsp Baking Powder
- 1 cup Mozzarella Cheese
- ¼ cup Cream Cheese
- 1 Egg

PREPARATION:

1. Preheat oven to 400F.
2. Melt the two cheeses together in the microwave.
3. Blend the melted cheese together then stir in the egg.
4. Whisk together the almond flour, psyllium husk, and baking powder in a separate bowl.
5. Mix the dry ingredients into the cheese mixture until a dough is formed.
6. Divide the dough into 6 and roll each portion into a ball.
7. Arrange on a baking sheet lined with parchment and bake for 12 minutes.

2. Keto Sandwich Bread

||||||||||||||||||||||||||||||||||||||||||||||||||||||

With less than a gram of net carbs per serving(yup, 2 slices), you can pretty much grab that favorite sandwich anytime of the day. Perfect!

DETAILS:

- Preparation Time: 15 minutes
- Cooking Time: 40 min
- Serves: 8

NUTRITIONAL VALUES:

- Kcal per serve: 209
- Fat: 21 g. (89%)
- Protein: 5 g. (10%)
- Carbs: 1g. (1%)

INGREDIENTS:

- 2 cups Almond Flour
- 1 tsp Baking Powder
- ½ tsp Xanthan Gum
- ½ tsp Salt
- ¾ cup Melted Butter
- 6 Large Eggs

PREPARATION:

1. Preheat oven to 350F.
2. Whisk together almond flour, baking powder, xanthan gum, and salt in a bowl.
3. In a separate bowl, beat the eggs and gradually whisk in the melted butter.
4. Mix the dry mixture in.
5. Pour the batter into a loaf pan lined with parchment.
6. Bake for 40 minutes.
7. Cool for about 15 minutes before slicing.

3. Keto Cinnamon Rolls

||||||||||||||||||||||||||||||||||||||||||||||||

Perfectly fluffy and delicious! It's really unbelievable how these treats roll out so low in unwanted carbs.

DETAILS:

- Preparation Time: 15 min
- Cooking Time: 20 minutes
- Serves: 8

NUTRITIONAL VALUES:

- Kcal per serve: 339
- Fat: 34 g. (87%)
- Protein: 4 g. (5%)
- Carbs: 7 g. (8%)

INGREDIENTS:

- 1 cup Almond Flour
- ¼ cup Psyllium Husk Powder
- 1 tbsp Active Dry Yeast
- ¼ cup Erythritol
- 1 tbsp Xanthan Gum
- 1 tbsp Baking Powder
- 1 tsp Salt
- 1 tbsp Maple Syrup
- 3 tbsp Lukewarm Water
- ¼ cup Coconut Cream
- 2 tbsp Melted Butter
- *For the Filling:*
- ¼ cup Softened Butter
- ¼ cup Erythritol
- 2 tbsp Ground Cinnamon
- *For the Glaze:*
- ½ cup Cream Cheese
- ½ cup Butter
- ¼ cup Erythritol
- 1 tsp Vanilla Extract

PREPARATION:

1. Whisk together warm water, yeast, coconut cream, and maple syrup in a bowl. Leave for 5-10 minutes to let the yeast activate.
2. Whisk together almond flour, psyllium husk, erythritol, xanthan gum, baking powder, and salt in a separate bowl.
3. After the yeast has proofed, whisk in the eggs and butter.
4. Stir the dry mixture into the wet ingredients until a sticky dough is formed.
5. Cover your work station with cling film to prevent the dough from sticking.
6. For the filling, whisk together erythritol and cinnamon.
7. Working in batches, take 1/3 of the dough and spread it with your fingers into a rectangle approximately 8"x10".
8. Cut the dough into 3 portions.
9. Brush each portion with butter then sprinkle cinnamon sugar on top.
10. Roll each filled portion, lightly pressing with the hand.
11. Arrange the rolls on a tray lined with parchment, cover with a kitchen towel, and leave to rise for an hour.
12. Meanwhile, whisk all ingredients for the glaze until fluffy.
13. Once the dough has fully risen, bake for 20 minutes in an oven preheated to 400F.
14. Take the rolls out of the oven and brush with the prepared glaze.

4. Keto Bread Sticks

|||||||||||||||||||||||||||||||||||||||||||||||||||

Whether it be a hot bowl of savory zoodles or a hearty serving of creamy chowder, these low-carb bread sticks would inarguably make any meal much more enjoyable. And they're perfect for snacking too!

DETAILS:

- Preparation Time: 10 minutes
- Cooking Time: 12 min
- Serves: 12

NUTRITIONAL VALUES:

- Kcal per serve: 56
- Fat: 4 g. (72%)
- Protein: 3 g. (24%)
- Carbs: 1 g. (4%)

INGREDIENTS:

- ¾ cup Almond Flour
- 1 tbsp Psyllium Husk Powder
- 1 tsp Baking Powder
- 1 cup Shredded Mozzarella
- ¼ cup Cream Cheese
- 1 Egg

PREPARATION:

1. Preheat oven to 400F.
2. Melt the two cheeses together in the microwave.
3. Blend the melted cheese together then stir in the egg.
4. Whisk together the almond flour, psyllium husk, and baking powder in a separate bowl.
5. Mix the dry ingredients into the cheese mixture until a dough is formed.
6. Roll the dough flat in between two sheets of parchment.
7. With a pizza cutter, portion the flattened dough out into sticks.
8. Arrange on a baking sheet lined with parchment and bake for 12 minutes.

5. Keto Banana Loaf

||||||||||||||||||||||||||||||||||||||||||||||||||||||

Who can resist a warm, moist, and very aromatic slice of banana bread? Well, this one's low-carb, so munch away!

DETAILS:

- Preparation Time: 10 min
- Cooking Time: 1 hour
- Serves: 12

NUTRITIONAL VALUES:

- Kcal per serve: 192
- Fat: 17 g. (78%)
- Protein: 5 g. (10%)
- Carbs: 6 g. (12%)

INGREDIENTS:

- 2 cups Almond Flour
- ¼ cup Coconut Flour
- 1 tbsp Baking Powder
- 1 tbsp Cinnamon Powder
- ¼ tsp Salt
- ½ cup Chopped Walnuts
- ½ cup Butter
- ½ cup Erythritol
- 4 Large Eggs
- ¼ cup Almond Milk
- 1 tbsp Banana Extract

PREPARATION:

1. Preheat oven to 350F.
2. Mix together the almond butter, coconut flour, baking powder, cinnamon, and salt in a bowl.
3. In a separate bowl, cream the butter and erythritol. Beat in the eggs, banana extract, and milk.
4. Mix the dry ingredients into the wet mixture.
5. Fold in the chopped walnuts.
6. Scrape the batter into a loaf pan lined with parchment.
7. Bake for 50-60 minutes.
8. Allow to cool before slicing.

6. Keto English Muffins

|||||||||||||||||||||||||||||||||||||||||||||||||||

Simple and quick to prepare, no other keto-friendly bread could be more perfect for breakfast.
Cook up some bacon and eggs and you're all set for a long day!

DETAILS:

- Preparation Time: 5 min
- Cooking Time: 3 min
- Serves: 3

NUTRITIONAL VALUES:

- Kcal per serve: 173
- Fat: 16 g. (85%)
- Protein: 5 g. (13%)
- Carbs: 1 g. (3%)

INGREDIENTS:

- 2 tbsp Almond Flour
- ½ tsp Baking Powder
- ½ tsp Salt
- 2 Large Eggs
- 3 tbsp Butter

PREPARATION:

1. Whisk together almond flour, baking powder, and salt in a bowl.
2. Whisk in the eggs.
3. Heat butter in a non-stick pan.
4. Ladle in the batter and cook for 2-3 minutes per side.

7. Keto Biscuits

||||||||||||||||||||||||||||||||||||||||||||||||||

Smoky bacon bits and sharp cheddar in a warm, tender, and fluffy muffin. These alone are perfect for breakfast!

DETAILS:

- Preparation Time: 10 minutes
- Cooking Time: 10 min
- Serves: 12

NUTRITIONAL VALUES:

- Kcal per serve: 182
- Fat: 16 g. (76%)
- Protein: 7 g. (15%)
- Carbs: 4 g. (9%)

INGREDIENTS:

- 1.5 cups Almond Flour
- 1 tbsp Baking Powder
- ¼ tsp Salt
- ½ tsp Onion Powder
- ½ cup Cream Cheese
- ½ cup Shredded Cheddar
- ¼ cup Bacon Bits
- 2 Whole Eggs
- ¼ cup Melted Butter

PREPARATION:

1. Preheat oven to 450F.
2. Whisk together almond flour, baking powder, salt, and onion powder in a bowl.
3. In a separate bowl, mix together eggs, cream cheese, and butter.
4. Stir the mixture into the dry ingredients.
5. Fold in the shredded cheddar and bacon bits.
6. Divide the batter into a pre-greased muffin tin.
7. Bake for 10 minutes.

8. Keto Garlic Bread

||||||||||||||||||||||||||||||||||||||||||||||||

A highly recommended treat for all garlic lovers out there. These are honestly too addictive!

DETAILS:

- Preparation Time: 15 minutes
- Cooking Time: 12 min
- Serves: 12

NUTRITIONAL VALUES:

- Kcal per serve: 130
- Fat: 11 g. (72%)
- Protein: 5 g. (15%)
- Carbs: 4 g. (12%)

INGREDIENTS:

- 2 cups Almond Flour
- ½ tsp Salt
- 1 tsp Baking Powder
- 1 tsp Garlic Powder
- 1 Whole Egg
- ½ cup Mozzarella, shredded

For the Topping:

- 2 tbsp Melted Butter
- ½ tsp Garlic Powder
- 1 tbsp Chopped Parsley

PREPARATION:

1. Preheat oven to 400F.
2. Whisk together the almond flour, baking powder, salt, and garlic powder in a bowl.
3. Crack the egg in and mix well.
4. Stir in the cheese and gently knead into a dough.
5. Roll the dough flat in between two sheets of parchment.
6. With a pizza cutter, portion the flattened dough out into sticks.
7. Arrange on a baking sheet lined with parchment.
8. Mix all ingredients for the topping and brush on top of the dough.
9. Bake for 10-12 minutes.

9. Keto Aurora Toast

||||||||||||||||||||||||||||||||||||||||||||||||||

Butter, sugar, and cinnamon – a simple yet effective harmony of flavors. These toasts may just be the universal definition of breakfast.

DETAILS:

- Preparation Time: 10 minutes
- Cooking Time: 12 min
- Serves: 12

NUTRITIONAL VALUES:

- Kcal per serve: 106
- Fat: 9 g. (76%)
- Protein: 4 g. (17%)
- Carbs: 2 g. (7%)

INGREDIENTS:

- ¾ cup Almond Flour
- 1 tbsp Psyllium Husk Powder
- 1 tsp Baking Powder
- 1 cup Shredded Mozzarella
- ¼ cup Cream Cheese
- 1 Egg

For Topping:

- 2 tbsp Melted Butter
- 1 tsp Cinnamon
- ¼ cup Erythritol

PREPARATION:

1. Preheat oven to 400F.
2. Melt the two cheeses together in the microwave.
3. Blend the melted cheese together then stir in the egg.
4. Whisk together the almond flour, psyllium husk, and baking powder in a separate bowl.
5. Mix the dry ingredients into the cheese mixture until a dough is formed.
6. Roll the dough flat in between two sheets of parchment.
7. Brush flattened dough with melted butter and mixture of erythritol and powdered cinnamon.
8. With a pizza cutter, portion the flattened dough out into sticks.
9. Arrange on a baking sheet lined with parchment and bake for 12 minutes.

10. Keto Zucchini Bread

||||||||||||||||||||||||||||||||||||||||||||||||||||

A low-carb loaf that's packed with all the nutrients and fiber of zucchini. Excellent!

DETAILS:

- Preparation Time: 10 min
- Cooking Time: 1 hour
- Serves: 12

NUTRITIONAL VALUES:

- Kcal per serve: 83
- Fat: 7 g. (80%)
- Protein: 2 g. (13%)
- Carbs: 2 g. (6%)

INGREDIENTS:

- 2 cups Almond Flour
- ¼ cup Coconut Flour
- 1 tbsp Baking Powder
- ¼ tsp Salt
- ½ cup Grated Zucchini
- ½ cup Butter
- ¼ cup Erythritol
- 4 Large Eggs
- ¼ cup Almond Milk

PREPARATION:

1. Preheat oven to 350F.
2. Mix together the almond butter, coconut flour, baking powder, and salt in a bowl.
3. In a separate bowl, cream the butter and erythritol. Beat in the eggs and milk.
4. Mix the dry ingredients into the wet mixture.
5. Fold in the grated zucchini.
6. Scrape the batter into a loaf pan lined with parchment.
7. Bake for 50-60 minutes.
8. Allow to cool before slicing.

11. Keto Cloud Bread

||||||||||||||||||||||||||||||||||||||||||||||||

Fluffy bread with just 3 easy ingredients. With less than a gram of carbs per serving, wouldn't you call this recipe perfect?

DETAILS:

- Preparation Time: 15 minutes
- Cooking Time: 25 min
- Serves: 8

NUTRITIONAL VALUES:

- Kcal per serve: 98
- Fat: 8 g. (78%)
- Protein: 4 g. (19%)
- Carbs: 1 g. (4%)

INGREDIENTS:

- 3 Whole Eggs, separated
- ½ cup Cream Cheese
- ¼ tsp Salt

PREPARATION:

1. Preheat oven to 300F.
2. Combine egg whites and salt in a bowl. Whip into stiff peaks.
3. In a separate bowl, beat together the egg yolks and cream cheese.
4. Gently fold in the yolk mixture into the whipped egg whites.
5. Dollop the mixture onto a parchment-lined baking tray, creating about 8 portions.
6. Bake for 25 minutes.

12. Keto Bagels

||||||||||||||||||||||||||||||||||||||||||||||||||||

Craving for a bagel but feeling too guilty from all those unwanted calories from carbs? We've got a solution for that!

DETAILS:

- Preparation Time: 10 minutes
- Cooking Time: 15 min
- Serves: 6

NUTRITIONAL VALUES:

- Kcal per serve: 96
- Fat: 8 g. (70%)
- Protein: 5 g. (23%)
- Carbs: 2g. (7%)

INGREDIENTS:

- ¼ cup Almond Flour
- 1 tsp Baking Powder
- ¼ tsp Salt
- 1 cup Shredded Mozzarella
- 2 tbsp Cream Cheese

PREPARATION:

1. Preheat oven to 425F.
2. Whisk together almond flour, baking powder, and salt in a bowl.
3. Melt both cheeses together in the microwave.
4. Stir in the eggs then the dry mixture.
5. Divide the dough into six portions.
6. Roll each portion into a ball and shape into logs.
7. Fold both ends of each log together to form a bagel.
8. Arrange on a baking sheet lined with parchment.
9. Bake for 15 minutes.

13. Keto Pull-Apart Rolls

||||||||||||||||||||||||||||||||||||||||||||||||||||

These rolls are unbelievably fluffy and chewy to think that they're actually free of gluten. Going keto with this recipe at hand does feel like cheating.

DETAILS:

- Preparation Time: 15 min
- Cooking Time: 20 minutes
- Serves: 8

NUTRITIONAL VALUES:

- Kcal per serve: 162
- Fat: 15 g. (79%)
- Protein: 3 g. (7%)
- Carbs: 6 g. (14%)

INGREDIENTS:

- 1 cup Almond Flour
- ¼ cup Psyllium Husk Powder
- 1 tbsp Active Dry Yeast
- ¼ cup Erythritol
- 1 tbsp Xanthan Gum
- 1 tbsp Baking Powder
- 1 tsp Salt
- 1 tbsp Maple Syrup
- 3 tbsp Lukewarm Water
- ¼ cup Milk
- 2 tbsp Melted Butter
- ¼ cup Butter, for brushing

PREPARATION:

1. Whisk together warm water, yeast, milk, and maple syrup in a bowl. Leave for 5-10 minutes to let the yeast activate.
2. Whisk together almond flour, psyllium husk, erythritol, xanthan gum, baking powder, and salt in a separate bowl.
3. After the yeast has proofed, whisk in the eggs and 2 tablespoons of butter.
4. Stir the dry mixture into the wet ingredients until a sticky dough is formed.
5. Divide the dough into 8 portions and roll each portion into a ball.
6. Arrange the balls of dough on a tray lined with parchment, cover with a kitchen towel, and leave to rise for an hour.
7. Once the dough has fully risen, brush with melted butter.
8. Bake for 20 minutes in an oven preheated to 400F.

14. Keto Cauliflower Bread

||||||||||||||||||||||||||||||||||||||||||||||||||||||

Warm, moist, delicious. These cauliflower bread bites do make for an excellent on-the-go snack.

DETAILS:

- Preparation Time: 10 min
- Cooking Time: 10 min
- Serves: 12

NUTRITIONAL VALUES:

- Kcal per serve: 188
- Fat: 17 g. (79%)
- Protein: 5 g. (11%)
- Carbs: 5 g. (10%)

INGREDIENTS:

- 2 cups Almond Flour
- 1 tbsp Baking Powder
- ¼ tsp Salt
- ½ cup Cauliflower, riced
- ½ cup Butter
- 4 Large Eggs
- ¼ cup Almond Milk

PREPARATION:

1. Preheat oven to 350F.
2. Mix together the almond butter, baking powder, and salt in a bowl.
3. In a separate bowl, beat together the eggs, butter, and milk.
4. Mix the dry ingredients into the wet mixture.
5. Fold in the cauliflower.
6. Divide the batter into a pre-greased muffin tin.
7. Bake for 10 minutes.

15. Keto Cheese Bread

||||||||||||||||||||||||||||||||||||||||||||||

Fluffy, yummy, and extremely cheesy! It's a good thing these go low on carbs. . . they're just that hard to resist.

DETAILS:

- Preparation Time: 10 minutes
- Cooking Time: 25 min
- Serves: 6

NUTRITIONAL VALUES:

- Kcal per serve: 203
- Fat: 16 g. (70%)
- Protein: 9 g. (18%)
- Carbs: 6 g. (12%)

INGREDIENTS:

- 1 cup Almond Flour
- 1 tsp Baking Powder
- ¼ tsp Salt
- 1/3 cup Milk
- 2 large Whole Eggs
- 1/3 cup Cream Cheese, softened
- ½ cup Grated Parmesan

PREPARATION:

1. Preheat oven to 350F.
2. Whisk together almond flour, baking powder, and salt in a bowl.
3. Beat eggs and cream cheese in a separate bowl. Gradually stir in the milk.
4. Stir the wet mixture into the dry ingredients.
5. Fold in the grated parmesan.
6. Coat a 6-hole muffin tin with non-stick spray.
7. Divide the batter into the pan and bake for 25 minutes.

16. Keto Mug Bread

|||||||||||||||||||||||||||||||||||||||||||||||||

So you're doing good so far into the keto diet, craving for bread, and got no baking skills. If you've at least got a microwave then you're not in that bad of a situation after all.

DETAILS:

- Preparation Time: 2 min
- Cooking Time: 2 min
- Serves: 1

NUTRITIONAL VALUES:

- Kcal per serve: 416
- Fat: 37 g. (77%)
- Protein: 15 g. (15%)
- Carbs: 8 g. (8%)

INGREDIENTS:

- 1/3 cup Almond Flour
- ½ tsp Baking Powder
- ¼ tsp Salt
- 1 Whole Egg
- 1 tbsp Melted Butter

PREPARATION:

1. Mix all ingredients in a microwave-safe mug.
2. Microwave for 90 seconds.
3. Cool for 2 minutes.

17. Keto Blender Buns

Blend it and bake it. Yup, it's that easy!

DETAILS:

- Preparation Time: 5 minutes
- Cooking Time: 25 min
- Serves: 6

NUTRITIONAL VALUES:

- Kcal per serve: 200
- Fat: 18 g. (79%)
- Protein: 8 g. (16%)
- Carbs: 2 g. (5%)

INGREDIENTS:

- 4 Whole Eggs
- ¼ cup Melted Butter
- ½ tsp Salt
- ½ cup Almond Flour
- 1 tsp Italian Spice Mix

PREPARATION:

1. Preheat oven to 425F.
2. Pulse all ingredients in a blender.
3. Divide batter into a 6-hole muffin tin.
4. Bake for 25 minutes.

18. Keto Ciabatta

||||||||||||||||||||||||||||||||||||||||||||||||

Fluffy and very aromatic. This ciabatta is perfect with just about anything from your favorite cheese to that sumptuous stew for dinner.

DETAILS:

- Preparation Time: 1 hour
- Cooking Time: 30 minutes
- Serves: 8

NUTRITIONAL VALUES:

- Kcal per serve: 121
- Fat: 11 g. (79%)
- Protein: 3 g. (9%)
- Carbs: 4 g. (13%)

INGREDIENTS:

- 1 cup Almond Flour
- ¼ cup Psyllium Husk Powder
- ½ tsp Salt
- 1 tsp Baking Powder
- 3 tbsp Olive Oil
- 1 tsp Maple Syrup
- 1 tbsp Active Dry Yeast
- 1 cup Warm Water
- 1 tbsp Chopped Rosemary

PREPARATION:

1. In a bowl, stir together warm water, maple syrup, and yeast. Leave for 10 minutes.
2. In a separate bowl, whisk together almond flour, psyllium husk powder, salt, chopped rosemary, and baking powder.
3. Stir in the olive oil and yeast mixture into the dry ingredients until a smooth dough is formed.
4. Knead the dough until smooth.
5. Divide the dough into 2 and shape into buns.
6. Set both buns on a baking sheet lined with parchment. Leave to rise for an hour.
7. Bake for 30 minutes at 380F.

19. Keto Burger Buns

||||||||||||||||||||||||||||||||||||||||||||||

So, should going on a keto diet suggest that you should be havin' that juicy burger on anything other than a soft and warm bun, like a wedge of iceberg lettuce perhaps? No thanks. There's gotta be a more clever solution to that problem.

DETAILS:

- Preparation Time: 10 minutes
- Cooking Time: 12 min
- Serves: 6

NUTRITIONAL VALUES:

- Kcal per serve: 216
- Fat: 18 g. (73%)
- Protein: 10 g. (18%)
- Carbs: 5 g. (9%)

INGREDIENTS:

- 1 cup Almond Flour
- ¼ cup Psyllium Husk Powder
- 1 tsp Baking Powder
- 1 cup Mozzarella Cheese
- ¼ cup Cream Cheese
- 1 Egg
- 1.5 tbsp Sesame Seeds

PREPARATION:

1. Preheat oven to 400F.
2. Melt the two cheeses together in the microwave.
3. Blend the melted cheese together then stir in the egg.
4. Whisk together the almond flour, psyllium husk, and baking powder in a separate bowl.
5. Mix the dry ingredients into the cheese mixture until a dough is formed.
6. Divide the dough into 6 and roll each portion into a ball.
7. Top each ball with sesame seeds.
8. Arrange on a baking sheet lined with parchment and bake for 12 minutes.
9. Leave to cool for 10-15 minutes before slicing into halves.

20. Keto Pizza Crust

||||||||||||||||||||||||||||||||||||||||||||||||||||

We might all agree that if it ain't for that crust, a pizza may just be the perfect keto food. Well, this recipe's keeping it that way!

DETAILS:

- Preparation Time: 10 minutes
- Cooking Time: 6 min
- Serves: 8

NUTRITIONAL VALUES:

- Kcal per serve: 165
- Fat: 13 g. (70%)
- Protein: 9 g. (22%)
- Carbs: 3 g. (8%)

INGREDIENTS:

- 1 cup Almond Flour
- 2 cups Shredded Mozzarella
- 2 tbsp Cream Cheese
- pinch of Salt

PREPARATION:

1. Combine both cheeses in a bowl and melt in the microwave.
2. Stir then gradually knead in the salt and almond flour.
3. Roll out to flatten in between sheets of parchment.
4. Bake at 350F for 6 minutes.
5. Put choice of toppings on and bake for another 5-10 minutes.

<u>Flatbreads</u>

1. Coco-Cilantro Flatbread

|||||||||||||||||||||||||||||||||||||||||||||||||||

Extremely aromatic and savory flatbreads at only a gram of net carbs per piece. Now you've got something perfect to go with your favorite keto curry!

DETAILS:

- Preparation Time: 10 minutes
- Cooking Time: 15 min
- Serves: 6

NUTRITIONAL VALUES:

- Kcal per serve: 46
- Fat: 4 g. (84%)
- Protein: 1 g. (3%)
- Carbs: 1 g. (13%)

INGREDIENTS:

- ½ cup Coconut Flour
- 2 tbsp Flax Meal
- ¼ tsp Baking Soda
- pinch of Salt
- 1 tbsp Coconut Oil
- 2 tbsp Chopped Cilantro
- 1 cup Lukewarm Water

PREPARATION:

1. Whisk together the coconut flour, flax, baking soda, and salt in a bowl.
2. Add in the water, coconut oil, and chopped cilantro.
3. Knead until everything comes together into a smooth dough.
4. Leave to rest for about 15 minutes.
5. Divide the dough into 6 equal-sized portions.
6. Roll each portion into a ball, then flatten with a rolling pin in between sheets of parchment paper.
7. Refrigerate until ready to use.
8. To cook, heat in a non-stick pan for 2-3 minutes per side.

2. Almond Curry Naan

|||||||||||||||||||||||||||||||||||||||||||||||||||

A low-carb flatbread with a pronounced curry flavor. These are so good, you would want to snack on them alone.

DETAILS:

- Preparation Time: 15 minutes
- Cooking Time: 15 min
- Serves: 6

NUTRITIONAL VALUES:

- Kcal per serve: 67
- Fat: 6 g. (80%)
- Protein: 2 g. (9%)
- Carbs: 2 g. (11%)

INGREDIENTS:

- ½ cup Almond Flour
- 2 tbsp Psyllium Husk
- ¼ tsp Baking Soda
- pinch of Salt
- 1 tsp Curry Powder
- 1 tbsp Olive Oil
- 1 cup Lukewarm Water

PREPARATION:

1. Whisk together the almond flour, curry powder, psyllium husk, baking soda, and salt in a bowl.
2. Add in the water and olive oil.
3. Knead until everything comes together into a smooth dough.
4. Leave to rest for about 15 minutes.
5. Divide the dough into 6 equal-sized portions.
6. Roll each portion into a ball, then flatten with a rolling pin in between sheets of parchment paper.
7. Refrigerate until ready to use.
8. To cook, heat in a non-stick pan for 2-3 minutes per side.

3. Chili and Cheese Tortillas

||||||||||||||||||||||||||||||||||||||||||||||||||||||||

Smoky, cheesy, and subtly spicy tortillas with just a handful of ingredients. Perfect with a bowl of your favorite chili!

DETAILS:

- Preparation Time: 10 min
- Cooking Time: 20 minutes
- Serves: 6

NUTRITIONAL VALUES:

- Kcal per serve: 246
- Fat: 20 g. (70%)
- Protein: 10 g. (17%)
- Carbs: 8 g. (13%)

INGREDIENTS:

- ¾ cup Mozzarella Cheese
- 1 tbsp Cream Cheese
- 1 Egg
- 2 tbsp Almond Flour
- 1 tsp Paprika
- pinch of Red Chili Flakes

PREPARATION:

1. Melt both cheeses in a double boiler.
2. Take off the heat and leave to cool for a few minutes.
3. Stir in the remaining ingredients.
4. Divide the dough into 6 portions and flatten onto a baking tray lined with parchment.
5. Bake for 20 minutes at 350F.

4. Garlic-Parmesan Chapati

||||||||||||||||||||||||||||||||||||||||||||

The tried and tested flavor combo of pungent garlic and salty cheese in a low-carb flatbread. This recipe will surely make its way to your collection of staples.

DETAILS:

- Preparation Time: 15 minutes
- Cooking Time: 15 min
- Serves: 6

NUTRITIONAL VALUES:

- Kcal per serve: 146
- Fat: 16 g. (96%)
- Protein: 1 g. (2%)
- Carbs: 1 g. (2%)

INGREDIENTS:

- ¾ cup Almond Flour
- 2 tbsp Psyllium Husk Powder
- ½ tsp Baking Powder
- ½ tsp Salt
- 1 tsp Garlic Powder
- 2 tbsp Grated Parmesan
- ½ cup Melted Butter
- 2 cups Lukewarm Water

PREPARATION:

1. Whisk together the almond flour, garlic powder, grated parmesan, psyllium husk, baking soda, and salt in a bowl.
2. Add in the water and melted butter.
3. Knead until everything comes together into a smooth dough.
4. Leave to rest for about 15 minutes.
5. Divide the dough into 6 equal-sized portions.
6. Roll each portion into a ball, then flatten with a rolling pin in between sheets of parchment paper.
7. Refrigerate until ready to use.
8. To cook, heat in a non-stick pan for 2-3 minutes per side.

5. Avocado Flatbread

||||||||||||||||||||||||||||||||||||||||||||||||||

These come out unbelievably soft and pliable for a bread that's totally vegan! Feel free to sprinkle in your favorite herbs into the dough to make the recipe much more personal.

DETAILS:

- Preparation Time: 25 min
- Cooking Time: 5 min
- Serves: 6

NUTRITIONAL VALUES:

- Kcal per serve: 80
- Fat: 4 g. (42%)
- Protein: 3 g. (16%)
- Carbs: 8 g. (42%)

INGREDIENTS:

- 130 grams Mashed Avocado
- ¾ cup Chickpea Flour
- 1 tsp Cumin Powder
- ½ tsp Salt

PREPARATION:

1. Combine all ingredients in a bowl. Stir until mixture comes together into a dough.
2. Knead the dough briefly on a lightly floured surface.
3. Leave the dough to rest for 15 minutes.
4. Divide the dough into four portions.
5. Take each portion of dough and flatten with a rolling pin.
6. Toast flatbread in a lightly oiled skillet for about 2 minutes per side.

5. Sun-Dried Tomato and Parsley Pitas

|||||||||||||||||||||||||||||||||||||||||||||||||||||||

Soft and perfectly chewy flatbreads with a unique twist on flavors. Yes, sun-dried tomatoes and fresh herbs can definitely be rolled into your favorite dough.

DETAILS:

- Preparation Time: 10 min
- Cooking Time: 20 minutes
- Serves: 6

NUTRITIONAL VALUES:

- Kcal per serve: 247
- Fat: 20 g. (70%)
- Protein: 11 g. (17%)
- Carbs: 8 g. (13%)

INGREDIENTS:

- ¾ cup Mozzarella Cheese
- 1 tbsp Cream Cheese
- 1 Egg
- 2 tbsp Almond Flour
- 1 tbsp Sun-Dried Tomato Pesto
- 1 tbsp Chopped Parsley

PREPARATION:

1. Melt both cheeses in a double boiler.
2. Take off the heat and leave to cool for a few minutes.
3. Stir in the remaining ingredients.
4. Divide the dough into 6 portions and flatten onto a baking tray lined with parchment.
5. Bake for 20 minutes at 350F.

7. Onion Roti

|||||||||||||||||||||||||||||||||||||||||||||||||

Another keto adaptation of the well-loved Indian flatbread. This one's infused with the natural sweetness of onions and the nutty flavor of coconuts.

DETAILS:

- Preparation Time: 10 minutes
- Cooking Time: 15 min
- Serves: 6

NUTRITIONAL VALUES:

- Kcal per serve: 57
- Fat: 6 g. (85%)
- Protein: 1 g. (2%)
- Carbs: 2 g. (13%)

INGREDIENTS:

- ¾ cup Coconut Flour
- 2 tbsp Xanthan Gum
- ¼ tsp Baking Soda
- pinch of Salt
- 1 tsp Onion Powder
- 1 tbsp Olive Oil
- 1 cup Lukewarm Water

PREPARATION:

1. Whisk together the coconut flour, onion powder, xanthan gum, baking soda, and salt in a bowl.
2. Add in the water and olive oil.
3. Knead until everything comes together into a smooth dough.
4. Leave to rest for about 15 minutes.
5. Divide the dough into 6 equal-sized portions.
6. Roll each portion into a ball, then flatten with a rolling pin in between sheets of parchment paper.
7. Refrigerate until ready to use.
8. To cook, heat in a non-stick pan for 2-3 minutes per side.

3. Butter Parsley Flatbread

||||||||||||||||||||||||||||||||||||||||||||||||||||

f herbed butter would surely work on pizza bases and bread sticks, why shouldn't it on a quick skillet flatbread? Perfect with just about anything for dinner.

DETAILS:

- Preparation Time: 10 minutes
- Cooking Time: 15 min
- Serves: 6

NUTRITIONAL VALUES:

- Kcal per serve: 207
- Fat: 21 g. (89%)
- Protein: 3 g. (5%)
- Carbs: 3 g. (6%)

INGREDIENTS:

- ¾ cup Almond Flour
- 2 tbsp Psyllium Husk Powder
- ½ tsp Baking Powder
- ½ tsp Salt
- 1 tsp Garlic Powder
- 1 tbsp Chopped Parsley
- ½ cup Melted Butter
- 2 cups Lukewarm Water

PREPARATION:

1. Whisk together the almond flour, garlic powder, chopped parsley, psyllium husk, baking soda, and salt in a bowl.
2. Add in the water and melted butter.
3. Knead until everything comes together into a smooth dough.
4. Leave to rest for about 15 minutes.
5. Divide the dough into 6 equal-sized portions.
6. Roll each portion into a ball, then flatten with a rolling pin in between sheets of parchment paper.
7. Refrigerate until ready to use.
8. To cook, heat in a non-stick pan for 2-3 minutes per side.

9. Spiced Soft Tacos

|||||||||||||||||||||||||||||||||||||||||||||||||||||

Finally, a low carb wrap to keep your favored taco fillings together. Given how soft and pliab
these tacos are, that idea will surely come in an instant.

DETAILS:

- Preparation Time: 10 minutes
- Cooking Time: 15 min
- Serves: 6

NUTRITIONAL VALUES:

- Kcal per serve: 68
- Fat: 6 g. (80%)
- Protein: 2 g. (9%)
- Carbs: 2 g. (11%)

INGREDIENTS:

- ½ cup Almond Flour
- 2 tbsp Psyllium Husk
- ¼ tsp Baking Soda
- pinch of Salt
- 1 tsp Paprika
- ½ tsp Ground Oregano
- 1 tbsp Avocado Oil
- 1 cup Lukewarm Water

PREPARATION:

1. Whisk together the almond flour, paprika, oregano, psyllium husk, baking soda, and salt in a bowl.
2. Add in the water and olive oil.
3. Knead until everything comes together into a smooth dough.
4. Leave to rest for about 15 minutes.
5. Divide the dough into 6 equal-sized portions.
6. Roll each portion into a ball, then flatten with a rolling pin in between sheets of parchment paper.
7. Refrigerate until ready to use.
8. To cook, heat in a non-stick pan for 2-3 minutes per side.

10. Spinach and Cheese Tortillas

|||||||||||||||||||||||||||||||||||||||||||||||||||

he rich flavor and cheese fortified with the healthy goodness of spinach. Perfect!

DETAILS:

- Preparation Time: 10 minutes
- Cooking Time: 20 min
- Serves: 6

NUTRITIONAL VALUES:

- Kcal per serve: 247
- Fat: 20 g. (70%)
- Protein: 11 g. (17%)
- Carbs: 8 g. (13%)

INGREDIENTS:

- ¾ cup Mozzarella Cheese
- 1 tbsp Cream Cheese
- 1 Egg
- 2 tbsp Almond Flour
- 1 tsp Paprika
- 2 tbsp Frozen Spinach, finely chopped

PREPARATION:

1. Melt both cheeses in a double boiler.
2. Take off the heat and leave to cool for a few minutes.
3. Stir in the remaining ingredients.
4. Divide the dough into 6 portions and flatten onto a baking tray lined with parchment.
5. Bake for 20 minutes at 350F.

Muffins & Cupcakes

1. Blueberry and Cream Cheese Muffins

||||||||||||||||||||||||||||||||||||||||||||||||

The classic blueberry cheesecake made into a keto-friendly muffin. Nothing else can be more inviting than these warm treats.

DETAILS:

- Preparation Time: 10 minutes
- Cooking Time: 25 min
- Serves: 6

NUTRITIONAL VALUES:

- Kcal per serve: 181
- Fat: 14 g. (69%)
- Protein: 7 g. (14%)
- Carbs: 8 g. (17%)

INGREDIENTS:

- 1 cup Almond Flour
- 1 tsp Baking Powder
- ¼ tsp Salt
- ½ cup Erythritol
- 1/3 cup Milk
- 2 large Whole Eggs
- 1/3 cup Cream Cheese, softened
- 1 cup Frozen Blueberries

PREPARATION:

1. Preheat oven to 350F.
2. Whisk together almond flour, baking powder, and salt in a bowl.
3. Beat eggs, erythritol, and cream cheese in a separate bowl. Gradually stir in the milk.
4. Stir the wet mixture into the dry ingredients.
5. Fold in the blueberries.
6. Coat a 6-hole muffin pan with non-stick spray.
7. Divide the batter into the pan and bake for 25 minutes.

2. Ham and Parmesan Muffins

||||||||||||||||||||||||||||||||||||||||||||||||||

The smokiness of ham and the sharp flavor of parmesan in a ready-to-go muffin. Perfect for breakfast or for anytime-of-the-day snacking.

DETAILS:

- Preparation Time: 10 minutes
- Cooking Time: 25 min
- Serves: 6

NUTRITIONAL VALUES:

- Kcal per serve: 230
- Fat: 18 g. (68%)
- Protein: 12 g. (21%)
- Carbs: 7 g. (12%)

INGREDIENTS:

- 1 cup Almond Flour
- 1 tsp Baking Powder
- ¼ tsp Salt
- ½ cup Erythritol
- 1/3 cup Milk
- 2 large Whole Eggs
- 1/3 cup Cream Cheese, softened
- ½ cup Grated Parmesan
- ½ cup Chopped Farmer's Ham

PREPARATION:

1. Preheat oven to 350F.
2. Whisk together almond flour, baking powder, and salt in a bowl.
3. Beat eggs, erythritol, and cream cheese in a separate bowl. Gradually stir in the milk.
4. Stir the wet mixture into the dry ingredients.
5. Fold in the chopped ham and grated parmesan.
6. Coat a 6-hole muffin pan with non-stick spray.
7. Divide the batter into the pan and bake for 25 minutes.

3. Cheddar Jalapeno Muffins

ounds familiar? Yes, the rich and perfectly tangy flavor of cheddar combined with the fruity int of jalapenos go perfectly well in a freshly baked goodies too!

DETAILS:

- Preparation Time: 10 minutes
- Cooking Time: 25 min
- Serves: 6

NUTRITIONAL VALUES:

- Kcal per serve: 228
- Fat: 20 g. (74%)
- Protein: 10 g. (18%)
- Carbs: 5 g. (9%)

INGREDIENTS:

- 1 cup Almond Flour
- 1 tsp Baking Powder
- ¼ tsp Salt
- ½ cup Erythritol
- 1/3 cup Milk
- 2 large Whole Eggs
- 1/3 cup Cream Cheese, softened
- 2/3 cup Shredded Cheddar Cheese
- 1 tbsp minced Jalapenos

PREPARATION:

1. Preheat oven to 350F.
2. Whisk together almond flour, baking powder, and salt in a bowl.
3. Beat eggs, erythritol, and cream cheese in a separate bowl. Gradually stir in the milk.
4. Stir the wet mixture into the dry ingredients.
5. Fold in the cheddar and jalapenos.
6. Coat a 6-hole muffin pan with non-stick spray.
7. Divide the batter into the pan and bake for 25 minutes.

4. Chocolate Zucchini Muffins

||||||||||||||||||||||||||||||||||||||||||||||||||

What better way to sneak in those veggies to your kids' diet? An irresistible chocolate muffin will surely do the trick.

DETAILS:

- Preparation Time: 10 minutes
- Cooking Time: 25 min
- Serves: 6

NUTRITIONAL VALUES:

- Kcal per serve: 280
- Fat: 26 g. (80%)
- Protein: 8 g. (10%)
- Carbs: 9 g. (10%)

INGREDIENTS:

- 1 cup Almond Flour
- 1 tsp Baking Powder
- ½ cup Unsweetened Cocoa Powder
- ¼ tsp Salt
- 1 cup Erythritol
- ¾ cup Buttermilk
- 2 large Whole Eggs
- 1 stick Butter, softened
- 1 cup Grated Zucchini

PREPARATION:

1. Preheat oven to 350F.
2. Whisk together almond flour, cocoa powder, baking powder, and salt in a bowl.
3. Cream butter and erythritol in a separate bowl. Beat in the eggs then gradually stir in the milk.
4. Stir the wet mixture into the dry ingredients.
5. Fold in the grated zucchini.
6. Coat a 6-hole muffin pan with non-stick spray.
7. Divide the batter into the pan and bake for 25 minutes.

5. Broccoli and Cheese Muffins

||||||||||||||||||||||||||||||||||||||||||||||||||

Makin' the well-loved cheese muffin even better with all the nutritional value of broccoli. A truly nutrient dense snack for the whole family.

DETAILS:

- Preparation Time: 10 minutes
- Cooking Time: 25 min
- Serves: 6

NUTRITIONAL VALUES:

- Kcal per serve: 167
- Fat: 14 g. (71%)
- Protein: 7 g. (16%)
- Carbs: 5 g. (13%)

INGREDIENTS:

- 1 cup Almond Flour
- 1 tsp Baking Powder
- ¼ tsp Salt
- ½ cup Erythritol
- 1/3 cup Milk
- 2 large Whole Eggs
- 1/3 cup Cream Cheese, softened
- 1 cup Broccoli, finely chopped

PREPARATION:

1. Preheat oven to 350F.
2. Whisk together almond flour, baking powder, and salt in a bowl.
3. Beat eggs, cream cheese, and erythritol in a separate bowl. Gradually stir in the milk.
4. Stir the wet mixture into the dry ingredients.
5. Fold in the chopped broccoli.
6. Coat a 6-hole muffin pan with non-stick spray.
7. Divide the batter into the pan and bake for 25 minutes.

6. Carrot Cardamom Muffins

||||||||||||||||||||||||||||||||||||||||||||||||||

The fragrance of cardamom gives unique life to this adaptation of the famous carrot cake. Let these muffins fill your house with all but comforting aromas.

DETAILS:

- Preparation Time: 10 minutes
- Cooking Time: 25 min
- Serves: 6

NUTRITIONAL VALUES:

- Kcal per serve: 178
- Fat: 14 g. (70%)
- Protein: 7 g. (15%)
- Carbs: 7 g. (15%)

INGREDIENTS:

- 1 cup Almond Flour
- 1 tsp Baking Powder
- ¼ tsp Salt
- ½ tsp Ground Cardamom
- ½ cup Erythritol
- 1/3 cup Milk
- 1 tsp Vanilla Extract
- 2 large Whole Eggs
- 1/3 cup Cream Cheese, softened
- 1 cup Grated Carrots

PREPARATION:

1. Preheat oven to 350F.
2. Whisk together almond flour, baking powder, and salt in a bowl.
3. Beat eggs, cream cheese, and erythritol in a separate bowl. Gradually stir in the milk and vanilla extract.
4. Stir the wet mixture into the dry ingredients.
5. Fold in the grated carrots.
6. Coat a 6-hole muffin pan with non-stick spray.
7. Divide the batter into the pan and bake for 25 minutes.

7. Squash and Cinnamon Muffins

|||||||||||||||||||||||||||||||||||||||||||||||||

Cinnamon ups the natural sweetness of butternut squash in a beautifully moist muffin. Highly recommended!

DETAILS:

- Preparation Time: 10 minutes
- Cooking Time: 25 min
- Serves: 6

NUTRITIONAL VALUES:

- Kcal per serve: 179
- Fat: 14 g. (69%)
- Protein: 7 g. (15%)
- Carbs: 8 g. (17%)

INGREDIENTS:

- 1 cup Almond Flour
- 1 tsp Baking Powder
- ½ tsp Cinnamon Powder
- ¼ tsp Salt
- ½ cup Erythritol
- 1/3 cup Milk
- 2 large Whole Eggs
- 1/3 cup Cream Cheese, softened
- 1 cup Butternut Squash, grated

PREPARATION:

1. Preheat oven to 350F.
2. Whisk together almond flour, baking powder, cinnamon, and salt in a bowl.
3. Beat eggs, erythritol, vanilla extract, and cream cheese in a separate bowl. Gradually stir in the milk.
4. Stir the wet mixture into the dry ingredients.
5. Fold in the butternut squash.
6. Coat a 6-hole muffin pan with non-stick spray.
7. Divide the batter into the pan and bake for 25 minutes.

8. Keto Red Velvet Muffins

|||||||||||||||||||||||||||||||||||||||||||||||||||

Everybody simply loves a anything that comes with red velvet in the label. Why can't keto fan
enjoy just the same?

DETAILS:

- Preparation Time: 10 minutes
- Cooking Time: 25 min
- Serves: 6

NUTRITIONAL VALUES:

- Kcal per serve: 331
- Fat: 32 g. (84%)
- Protein: 8 g. (9%)
- Carbs: 7 g. (7%)

INGREDIENTS:

- 1.25 cup Almond Flour
- 2 tbsp Unsweetened Cocoa Powder
- 1 tsp Baking Powder
- ¼ tsp Salt
- ½ cup Erythritol
- 1/3 cup Milk
- ½ cup Melted Butter
- 1.5 tsp Red Food Coloring
- 2 large Whole Eggs
- 1/3 cup Cream Cheese, softened

PREPARATION:

1. Preheat oven to 350F.
2. Whisk together almond flour, cocoa powder, baking powder, and salt in a bowl.
3. Beat eggs, erythritol, cream cheese, butter, and food coloring in a separate bowl. Gradually stir in the milk.
4. Stir the wet mixture into the dry ingredients.
5. Coat a 6-hole muffin pan with non-stick spray.
6. Divide the batter into the pan and bake for 25 minutes.

). Coffee Butter Muffins

he comforting mood and feel of early mornings in a freshly baked muffin. Now you can enjoy reakfast anytime of the day.

DETAILS:

- Preparation Time: 10 minutes
- Cooking Time: 25 min
- Serves: 6

NUTRITIONAL VALUES:

- Kcal per serve: 376
- Fat: 37 g. (85%)
- Protein: 8 g. (8%)
- Carbs: 8 g. (7%)

INGREDIENTS:

- 1.5 cups Almond Flour
- 1 tsp Instant Coffee
- 1 tsp Cinnamon Powder
- 1 tsp Baking Powder
- ¼ tsp Salt
- ½ cup Erythritol
- 1/3 cup Milk
- 2 large Whole Eggs
- ¾ cup Butter, softened

PREPARATION:

1. Preheat oven to 350F.
2. Whisk together almond flour, instant coffee, cinnamon, baking powder, and salt in a bowl.
3. Beat eggs, butter, and erythritol in a separate bowl. Gradually stir in the milk.
4. Stir the wet mixture into the dry ingredients.
5. Coat a 6-hole muffin pan with non-stick spray.
6. Divide the batter into the pan and bake for 25 minutes.

10. Choco Peanut Butter Muffins

||||||||||||||||||||||||||||||||||||||||||||||||||||||

Put together chocolate and peanut butter in a treat and anyone would surely give in. A richly flavored muffin that's unbelievably keto-friendly.

DETAILS:

- Preparation Time: 10 minutes
- Cooking Time: 25 min
- Serves: 6

NUTRITIONAL VALUES:

- Kcal per serve: 210
- Fat: 17 g. (69%)
- Protein: 10 g. (17%)
- Carbs: 8 g. (15%)

INGREDIENTS:

- 1 cup Almond Flour
- 1 tsp Baking Powder
- ¼ tsp Salt
- ½ cup Erythritol
- 1/3 cup Milk
- 2 large Whole Eggs
- 1 tsp Vanilla Extract
- 1/3 cup Peanut Butter
- 1 cup Sugar-Free Chocolate Chips

PREPARATION.

1. Preheat oven to 350F.
2. Whisk together almond flour, baking powder, and salt in a bowl.
3. Beat eggs, peanut butter, vanilla, and erythritol in a separate bowl. Gradually stir in the milk.
4. Stir the wet mixture into the dry ingredients.
5. Fold in the chocolate chips.
6. Coat a 6-hole muffin pan with non-stick spray.
7. Divide the batter into the pan and bake for 25 minutes.

1. Lemon Butter Cupcakes

||||||||||||||||||||||||||||||||||||||||||||||||||||||

oft and moist butter cupcakes with a bright hint of citrus. Best enjoyed when hot!

DETAILS:

- Preparation Time: 10 minutes
- Cooking Time: 25 min
- Serves: 6

NUTRITIONAL VALUES:

- Kcal per serve: 306
- Fat: 29 g. (82%)
- Protein: 8 g. (9%)
- Carbs: 7 g. (8%)

INGREDIENTS:

- 1.5 cups Almond Flour
- 1.5 tsp Baking Powder
- ¼ tsp Salt
- ½ cup Erythritol
- 1/3 cup Milk
- 2 large Whole Eggs
- 1 stick Butter, softened
- 2 tsp Lemon Zest

PREPARATION:

1. Preheat oven to 350F.
2. Whisk together almond flour, baking powder, and salt in a bowl.
3. Beat eggs, butter, and erythritol in a separate bowl. Gradually stir in the milk.
4. Stir the wet mixture into the dry ingredients.
5. Fold in the lemon zest.
6. Coat a 6-hole muffin pan with non-stick spray.
7. Divide the batter into the pan and bake for 25 minutes.

12. Three-Cheese Cupcakes

|||||||||||||||||||||||||||||||||||||||||||||||||||

Treat the senses with three cheeses of distinct flavor profiles. These cupcakes are simply delicious!

DETAILS:

- Preparation Time: 10 minutes
- Cooking Time: 25 min
- Serves: 6

NUTRITIONAL VALUES:

- Kcal per serve: 224
- Fat: 18 g. (72%)
- Protein: 10 g. (18%)
- Carbs: 6 g. (10%)

INGREDIENTS:

- 1 cup Almond Flour
- 1 tsp Baking Powder
- ¼ tsp Salt
- ½ cup Erythritol
- 1/3 cup Milk
- 2 large Whole Eggs
- 1/3 cup Cream Cheese, softened
- ½ cup Grated Cheddar
- ¼ cup Grated Parmesan

PREPARATION:

1. Preheat oven to 350F.
2. Whisk together almond flour, baking powder, and salt in a bowl.
3. Beat eggs, erythritol, and cream cheese in a separate bowl. Gradually stir in the milk.
4. Stir the wet mixture into the dry ingredients.
5. Fold in the cheddar and parmesan.
6. Coat a 6-hole muffin pan with non-stick spray.
7. Divide the batter into the pan and bake for 25 minutes.

3. Cinnamon Sugar Cupcakes

Simple yet effectively inviting. It's just amazing how two basic ingredients can work in so much harmony.

DETAILS:

- Preparation Time: 10 minutes
- Cooking Time: 25 min
- Serves: 6

NUTRITIONAL VALUES:

- Kcal per serve: 306
- Fat: 29 g. (82%)
- Protein: 8 g. (9%)
- Carbs: 7 g. (8%)

INGREDIENTS:

- 1.5 cups Almond Flour
- 1.5 tsp Baking Powder
- ¼ tsp Salt
- ½ tsp Cinnamon
- ½ cup Erythritol
- 1/3 cup Milk
- 2 large Whole Eggs
- 1 stick Butter, softened
- 2 tsp Lemon Zest

PREPARATION:

1. Preheat oven to 350F.
2. Whisk together almond flour, baking powder, cinnamon, and salt in a bowl.
3. Beat eggs, butter, and erythritol in a separate bowl. Gradually stir in the milk.
4. Stir the wet mixture into the dry ingredients.
5. Coat a 6-hole muffin pan with non-stick spray.
6. Divide the batter into the pan and bake for 25 minutes.

14. Strawberry Cream Cheese Cupcakes

||||||||||||||||||||||||||||||||||||||||||||||

Feel the slight tanginess of fresh strawberries cut perfectly through the richness of cream cheese in these delicious cupcakes. A real treat for any palate.

DETAILS:

- Preparation Time: 10 minutes
- Cooking Time: 25 min
- Serves: 6

NUTRITIONAL VALUES:

- Kcal per serve: 181
- Fat: 14 g. (68%)
- Protein: 7 g. (15%)
- Carbs: 9 g. (18%)

INGREDIENTS:

- 1 cup Almond Flour
- 1 tsp Baking Powder
- ¼ tsp Salt
- ½ cup Erythritol
- 1/3 cup Milk
- 2 large Whole Eggs
- 1/3 cup Cream Cheese, softened
- 1 cup Frozen Strawberries, diced

PREPARATION:

1. Preheat oven to 350F.
2. Whisk together almond flour, baking powder, and salt in a bowl.
3. Beat eggs, erythritol, and cream cheese in a separate bowl. Gradually stir in the milk.
4. Stir the wet mixture into the dry ingredients.
5. Fold in the strawberries.
6. Coat a 6-hole muffin pan with non-stick spray.
7. Divide the batter into the pan and bake for 25 minutes.

5. Coco-Blueberry Cupcakes

||||||||||||||||||||||||||||||||||||||||||||||||||||||

The deep nutty flavor of coconut and sweetness of blueberries come out distinct in these cupcakes. Definitely a must-try.

DETAILS:

- Preparation Time: 10 minutes
- Cooking Time: 25 min
- Serves: 6

NUTRITIONAL VALUES:

- Kcal per serve: 312
- Fat: 30 g. (84%)
- Protein: 6 g. (8%)
- Carbs: 7 g. (9%)

INGREDIENTS:

- 1 cup Almond Flour
- 1/2 cup Coconut Flour
- 1 tbsp Flax Meal
- 1 tsp Baking Powder
- ¼ tsp Salt
- ½ cup Erythritol
- 1/3 cup Milk
- 2 large Whole Eggs
- ½ cup Frozen Blueberries
- ½ cup Coconut Oil

PREPARATION:

1. Preheat oven to 350F.
2. Whisk together almond flour, coconut flour, baking powder, and salt in a bowl.
3. Beat eggs, coconut oil, and erythritol in a separate bowl. Gradually stir in the milk.
4. Stir the wet mixture into the dry ingredients.
5. Fold in the blueberries.
6. Coat a 6-hole muffin pan with non-stick spray.
7. Divide the batter into the pan and bake for 25 minutes.

16. Choco-Hazelnut Cupcakes

||||||||||||||||||||||||||||||||||||||||||||||||||

Hazelnuts add extra richness to these dark chocolate cupcakes. Some treats are simply meant to be savored.

DETAILS:

- Preparation Time: 10 minutes
- Cooking Time: 25 min
- Serves: 6

NUTRITIONAL VALUES:

- Kcal per serve: 318
- Fat: 29 g. (79%)
- Protein: 9 g. (10%)
- Carbs: 9 g. (10%)

INGREDIENTS:

- 1.25 cup Almond Flour
- ¼ cup Unsweetened Cocoa Powder
- 1.5 tsp Baking Powder
- ¼ tsp Salt
- ½ cup Erythritol
- 1/3 cup Milk
- 2 large Whole Eggs
- 1 tsp Vanilla Extract
- 1/3 cup Hazelnut Butter
- ½ cup Sugar-Free Chocolate Chips
- ½ cup Hazelnuts, chopped

PREPARATION:

1. Preheat oven to 350F.
2. Whisk together almond flour, cocoa powder, baking powder, and salt in a bowl.
3. Beat eggs, hazelnut butter, vanilla, and erythritol in a separate bowl. Gradually stir in the milk.
4. Stir the wet mixture into the dry ingredients.
5. Fold in the chocolate chips and hazelnuts.
6. Coat a 6-hole muffin pan with non-stick spray.
7. Divide the batter into the pan and bake for 25 minutes.

.7. Cheddar and Spinach Cupcakes

||||||||||||||||||||||||||||||||||||||||||||||

Healthy spinach cakes flavored with rich and perfectly sharp cheddar cheese. Simply excellent!

DETAILS:

- Preparation Time: 10 minutes
- Cooking Time: 25 min
- Serves: 6

NUTRITIONAL VALUES:

- Kcal per serve: 209
- Fat: 17 g. (73%)
- Protein: 9 g. (17%)
- Carbs: 5 g. (10%)

INGREDIENTS:

- 1 cup Almond Flour
- 1 tsp Baking Powder
- ¼ tsp Salt
- ½ cup Erythritol
- 1/3 cup Milk
- 2 large Whole Eggs
- 1/3 cup Cream Cheese, softened
- ½ cup Cheddar, shredded
- 1/3 cup Frozen Spinach, thawed and chopped

PREPARATION:

1. Preheat oven to 350F.
2. Whisk together almond flour, baking powder, and salt in a bowl.
3. Beat eggs, cream cheese, and erythritol in a separate bowl. Gradually stir in the milk.
4. Stir the wet mixture into the dry ingredients.
5. Fold in the cheddar and spinach.
6. Coat a 6-hole muffin pan with non-stick spray.
7. Divide the batter into the pan and bake for 25 minutes.

18. Mango-Cayenne Cupcakes

||||||||||||||||||||||||||||||||||||||||||||||

The fragrance and natural pleasing sweetness of ripe mangoes spiked up just right with a touch of cayenne. A truly unique experience awaits.

DETAILS:

- Preparation Time: 10 minutes
- Cooking Time: 25 min
- Serves: 6

NUTRITIONAL VALUES:

- Kcal per serve: 279
- Fat: 25 g. (79%)
- Protein: 8 g. (12%)
- Carbs: 7 g. (9%)

INGREDIENTS:

- 1 cup Almond Flour
- 1/2 cup Coconut Flour
- 1 tbsp Flax Meal
- ½ tsp Cayenne
- 1 tsp Baking Powder
- ¼ tsp Salt
- ½ cup Erythritol
- 1/3 cup Milk
- 2 large Whole Eggs
- ½ cup Sugar-Free Mango Jelly
- ½ cup Butter, softened

PREPARATION:

1. Preheat oven to 350F.
2. Whisk together almond flour, coconut flour, baking powder, flax meal, cayenne, and salt in a bowl.
3. Beat eggs, mango jelly, butter, and erythritol in a separate bowl. Gradually stir in the milk.
4. Stir the wet mixture into the dry ingredients.
5. Coat a 6-hole muffin pan with non-stick spray.
6. Divide the batter into the pan and bake for 25 minutes.

9. Lime and Vanilla Cupcakes

||||||||||||||||||||||||||||||||||||||||||||||

basic vanilla-flavored cupcakes lifted with a hint of fresh lime. Satisfying and fresh with every bite.

DETAILS:

- Preparation Time: 10 minutes
- Cooking Time: 25 min
- Serves: 6

NUTRITIONAL VALUES:

- Kcal per serve: 308
- Fat: 29 g. (82%)
- Protein: 8 g. (9%)
- Carbs: 7 g. (8%)

INGREDIENTS:

- 1.5 cups Almond Flour
- 1.5 tsp Baking Powder
- ¼ tsp Salt
- ½ cup Erythritol
- 1/3 cup Milk
- 2 large Whole Eggs
- 1 tsp Vanilla Extract
- 1 stick Butter, softened
- 2 tsp Lime Zest

PREPARATION:

1. Preheat oven to 350F.
2. Whisk together almond flour, baking powder, and salt in a bowl.
3. Beat eggs, butter, and erythritol, and vanilla in a separate bowl. Gradually stir in the milk.
4. Stir the wet mixture into the dry ingredients.
5. Fold in the lime zest.
6. Coat a 6-hole muffin pan with non-stick spray.
7. Divide the batter into the pan and bake for 25 minutes.

20. Chia Chocolate Cupcakes

||||||||||||||||||||||||||||||||||||||||||||||||||

Extremely moist chocolate cupcakes made far more healthy with the well-known benefits of chia. Yes, these seeds really do wonders in the kitchen!

DETAILS:

- Preparation Time: 10 minutes
- Cooking Time: 25 min
- Serves: 6

NUTRITIONAL VALUES:

- Kcal per serve: 257
- Fat: 23 g. (78%)
- Protein: 8 g. (12%)
- Carbs: 8 g. (10%)

INGREDIENTS:

- 1.25 cup Almond Flour
- ¼ cup Unsweetened Cocoa Powder
- 1.5 tsp Baking Powder
- ¼ tsp Salt
- ½ cup Erythritol
- 1/3 cup Milk
- 2 large Whole Eggs
- 1 tsp Vanilla Extract
- ½ cup Butter
- ½ cup Sugar-Free Chocolate Chips
- 2 tbsp Chia Seeds

PREPARATION:

1. Preheat oven to 350F.
2. Whisk together almond flour, cocoa powder, baking powder, and salt in a bowl.
3. Beat eggs, butter, vanilla, and erythritol in a separate bowl. Gradually stir in the milk.
4. Stir the wet mixture into the dry ingredients.
5. Fold in the chocolate chips and chia seeds.
6. Coat a 6-hole muffin pan with non-stick spray.
7. Divide the batter into the pan and bake for 25 minutes.

Cookies

1. Low-Carb Chocolate Chip Cookies

||||||||||||||||||||||||||||||||||||||||||||||||||

Quick and easy chocolate chip cookies that are unbelievably low in carbs! Definitely a sweet craving fix that won't get you out of ketosis.

DETAILS:

- Preparation Time: 10 minutes
- Cooking Time: 12 min
- Serves: 12

NUTRITIONAL VALUES:

- Kcal per serve: 148
- Fat: 14 g. (84%)
- Protein: 3 g. (8%)
- Carbs: 3 g. (8%)

INGREDIENTS:

- 1.5 cups Almond Flour
- ½ tsp Baking Powder
- ¼ tsp Salt
- 1 cup Sugar-Free Chocolate Chips
- 1 stick Butter, softened
- 1 tsp Vanilla Extract
- ½ cup Swerve Granular Sweetener
- 1 Whole Egg

PREPARATION:

1. Preheat oven to 350F.
2. Cream butter and sweetener with a mixer.
3. Mix in the egg and vanilla extract.
4. Whisk together the almond flour, baking powder, and salt in a separate bowl.
5. Mix the dry ingredients into the wet mixture.
6. Fold in the chocolate chips into the dough.
7. Scoop the dough into a baking sheet lined with parchment. Press slightly to flatten.
8. Bake for 12 minutes.

2. Keto Peanut Butter Cookies

||||||||||||||||||||||||||||||||||||||||||||||||||||||

xcellently chewy peanut butter cookies with just 3 ingredients. And with just 2 grams of net arbs per serving, what's not to like?

DETAILS:

- Preparation Time: 10 minutes
- Cooking Time: 12 min
- Serves: 12

NUTRITIONAL VALUES:

- Kcal per serve: 136
- Fat: 12 g. (79%)
- Protein: 5 g. (15%)
- Carbs: 2g. (6%)

INGREDIENTS:

- 1 cup Peanut Butter(sugar-free)
- ½ cup Erythritol
- 1 Whole Egg

PREPARATION:

1. Mix all ingredients a bowl until well combined.
2. Scoop the dough into a baking sheet lined with parchment. Press slightly to flatten.
3. Bake for 12 minutes.

3. Matcha Coconut Cookies

Nutty-flavored cookies with an earthy touch of matcha. The green tint from the tea even mak[es] these treats extra inviting.

DETAILS:

- Preparation Time: 10 min
- Cooking Time: 12 minutes
- Serves: 12

NUTRITIONAL VALUES:

- Kcal per serve: 112
- Fat: 12 g. (91%)
- Protein: 2 g. (5%)
- Carbs: 1 g. (4%)

INGREDIENTS:

- 1/3 cup Almond Flour
- 1/3 cup Coconut Flour
- 2 tbsp Matcha Powder
- ½ cup Swerve Granular Sweetener
- ½ tsp Baking Powder
- ½ cup Coconut Oil
- 1 Whole Egg

PREPARATION:

1. Whisk together the almond flour, coconut flour, sweetener, matcha, and baking powder i[n] a bowl.
2. Add in the egg and coconut oil. Mix until well combined.
3. Scoop the dough into a baking sheet lined with parchment. Press slightly to flatten.
4. Bake for 12 minutes.

4. Apricot and Cream Cheese Cookies

|||||||||||||||||||||||||||||||||||||||||||||||||||

erfect cream cheese cookies with the fruity hint and aroma of apricots. These are simply so elicious!

DETAILS:

- Preparation Time: 10 minutes
- Cooking Time: 12 min
- Serves: 15

NUTRITIONAL VALUES:

- Kcal per serve: 122
- Fat: 11 g. (79%)
- Protein: 4 g. (11%)
- Carbs: 3 g. (10%)

INGREDIENTS:

- 2 cups Almond Flour
- ½ tsp Baking Powder
- ¼ tsp Salt
- ¼ cup Cream Cheese, softened
- ¼ cup Sugar-Free Apricot Preserve
- ¼ cup Butter, softened
- 1 tsp Vanilla Extract
- ½ cup Swerve Granular Sweetener
- 1 Whole Egg

PREPARATION:

1. Preheat oven to 350F.
2. With a hand mixer, beat together the butter, cream cheese, sweetener, and apricot preserve until fluffy.
3. Mix in the egg and vanilla extract.
4. Whisk together the almond flour, baking powder, and salt in a separate bowl.
5. Mix the dry ingredients into the wet mixture.
6. Scoop the dough into a baking sheet lined with parchment. Press slightly to flatten.
7. Bake for 12 minutes.

5. Almond Butter Cookies

|||||||||||||||||||||||||||||||||||||||||||||||||||||

Extremely fragrant cookies that will surely satisfy any sweet craving. With its perfect balance of macros, these will keep you on track within a ketogenic diet.

DETAILS:

- Preparation Time: 10 min
- Cooking Time: 12 min
- Serves: 12

NUTRITIONAL VALUES:

- Kcal per serve: 159
- Fat: 14 g. (75%)
- Protein: 5 g. (13%)
- Carbs: 5 g. (12%)

INGREDIENTS:

- 1 cup Almond Butter
- ¼ cup Coconut Flour
- ½ cup Erythritol
- ¼ cup Slivered Almonds
- 1 Whole Egg
- 1 tsp Vanilla Extract

PREPARATION:

1. Preheat oven to 350F.
2. Mix together the almond butter, coconut flour, erythritol, vanilla, and egg in a bowl until well combined.
3. Fold in the slivered almonds.
4. Scoop the dough into a baking sheet lined with parchment. Press slightly to flatten.
5. Bake for 12 minutes.

6. Choco Hazelnut Butter Cookies

|||||||||||||||||||||||||||||||||||||||||||||||||||||||

The perfect harmony of bittersweet chocolate and rich hazelnuts in a low-carb cookie! This is sure to please anyone with a sweet tooth.

DETAILS:

- Preparation Time: 10 min
- Cooking Time: 12 min
- Serves: 12

NUTRITIONAL VALUES:

- Kcal per serve: 168
- Fat: 8 g. (95%)
- Protein: 1 g. (3%)
- Carbs: 2 g. (2%)

INGREDIENTS:

- 1 cup Hazelnut Butter
- ¼ cup Unsweetened Cocoa Powder
- ½ cup Erythritol
- ¼ cup Sugar-Free Chocolate Chips
- 1 Whole Egg
- ¼ cup Almond Milk
- 1 tsp Vanilla Extract

PREPARATION:

1. Preheat oven to 350F.
2. Mix together the hazelnut butter, cocoa powder, and erythritol in a bowl until well combined.
3. Stir in the egg and vanilla extract.
4. Add in milk a tablespoon at a time.
5. Fold in the chocolate chips.
6. Scoop the dough into a baking sheet lined with parchment. Press slightly to flatten.
7. Bake for 12 minutes.

7. Banana Walnut Cookies

||||||||||||||||||||||||||||||||||||||||||||||||||

Another keto adaptation of the well-loved Indian flatbread. This one's infused with the natur *sweetness of onions and the nutty flavor of coconuts.*

DETAILS:

- Preparation Time: 10 minutes
- Cooking Time: 12 min
- Serves: 12

NUTRITIONAL VALUES:

- Kcal per serve: 112
- Fat: 8 g. (61%)
- Protein: 3 g. (11%)
- Carbs: 8 g. (29%)

INGREDIENTS:

- 1.5 cups Almond Flour
- 1 cup Mashed Bananas
- ¼ cup Peanut Butter
- ¼ cup Walnuts, chopped

PREPARATION:

1. Preheat oven to 350F.
2. In a bowl, mix almond flour, mashed bananas, and peanut butter until well combined.
3. Fold in the walnuts into the dough.
4. Scoop the dough into a baking sheet lined with parchment. Press slightly to flatten.
5. Bake for 12 minutes.

3. Cinnamon Butter Cookies

||||||||||||||||||||||||||||||||||||||||||||||||||||

Warm aromatic cookies with a perfect balance of crisp and softness. Simple but highly recommended.

DETAILS:

- Preparation Time: 10 minutes
- Cooking Time: 12 min
- Serves: 12

NUTRITIONAL VALUES:

- Kcal per serve: 171
- Fat: 16 g. (82%)
- Protein: 4 g. (9%)
- Carbs: 3 g. (9%)

INGREDIENTS:

- 2 cups Almond Flour
- ¼ tsp Salt
- ½ tsp Cinnamon Powder
- 1 stick Butter, softened
- 1 tsp Vanilla Extract
- ½ cup Swerve Granular Sweetener
- 1 Whole Egg

PREPARATION:

1. Preheat oven to 350F.
2. Whisk together the almond flour, salt, cinnamon, and sweetener in a bowl.
3. Cut in the butter until mixture resembles a coarse meal.
4. Mix in the egg and vanilla extract.
5. Scoop the dough into a baking sheet lined with parchment. Press slightly to flatten.
6. Bake for 12 minutes.

9. Keto Ginger Cookies

||||||||||||||||||||||||||||||||||||||||||||||||||||||

Fill the kitchen with wonderful aromas that are sure to bring back happy memories. Then indulge into these warm and chewy cookies without any guilt.

DETAILS:

- Preparation Time: 10 minutes
- Cooking Time: 12 min
- Serves: 12

NUTRITIONAL VALUES:

- Kcal per serve: 137
- Fat: 13 g. (86%)
- Protein: 3 g. (7%)
- Carbs: 2 g. (7%)

INGREDIENTS:

- 1 cup Almond Flour
- ½ cup Coconut Flour
- ¼ tsp Salt
- ½ tsp Cinnamon Powder
- ½ tsp Ginger Powder
- ¼ tsp Ground Cloves
- 1 stick Butter, softened
- 1 tsp Vanilla Extract
- ½ cup Swerve Granular Sweetener
- 1 Whole Egg

PREPARATION:

1. Preheat oven to 350F.
2. Whisk together the almond flour, coconut flour, salt, cinnamon, ginger powder, cloves, and sweetener in a bowl.
3. Cut in the butter until mixture resembles a coarse meal.
4. Mix in the egg and vanilla extract.
5. Scoop the dough into a baking sheet lined with parchment. Press slightly to flatten.
6. Bake for 12 minutes.

0. Low-Carb Butter Pecan Cookies

||||||||||||||||||||||||||||||||||||||||||||||||||||

xtremely savory and crisp toasted pecans in a soft almond butter cookie. Doesn't that sound) delicious?

DETAILS:

- Preparation Time: 10 minutes
- Cooking Time: 12 min
- Serves: 15

NUTRITIONAL VALUES:

- Kcal per serve: 160
- Fat: 15 g. (83%)
- Protein: 3 g. (8%)
- Carbs: 3 g. (9%)

INGREDIENTS:

- 2 cups Almond Flour
- ½ tsp Baking Powder
- ¼ tsp Salt
- ½ cup Pecans, chopped
- 1 stick Butter, softened
- 1 tsp Vanilla Extract
- ½ cup Swerve Granular Sweetener
- 1 Whole Egg

PREPARATION:

1. Preheat oven to 350F.
2. Cream butter, sweetener with a mixer.
3. Mix in the egg and vanilla extract.
4. Whisk together the almond flour, baking powder, and salt in a separate bowl.
5. Mix the dry ingredients into the wet mixture.
6. Fold in the chopped pecans into the dough.
7. Scoop the dough into a baking sheet lined with parchment. Press slightly to flatten.
8. Bake for 12 minutes.

Pancakes

. Almond Banana Pancakes

|||||||||||||||||||||||||||||||||||||||||||||||||||

Start your day right with these light and fluffy banana pancakes. Everythin' else may be in a rush this time of the day, but definitely not those sugars!

DETAILS:

- Preparation Time: 10 minutes
- Cooking Time: 10 minutes
- Serves: 4

NUTRITIONAL VALUES:

- Kcal per serve: 235
- Fat: 17 g. (64%)
- Protein: 11 g. (21%)
- Carbs: 10 g. (16%)

INGREDIENTS:

- 1 Ripe Banana, mashed
- 4 Eggs
- 1/2 cup Almond Flour
- 2 tbsp Erythritol
- 1 tsp Baking Powder
- 1 tsp Ground Cinnamon

PREPARATION:

1. Whisk together almond flour, baking powder, and cinnamon in a bowl.
2. In a separate bowl, mix together mashed banana, eggs, and erythritol.
3. Gradually fold in the dry ingredients into the wet mixture.
4. Preheat a skillet and coat with non-stick spray.
5. Ladle in the batter and cook for 1-2 minutes per side.

2. Jalapeno and Cream Cheese Pancakes

||||||||||||||||||||||||||||||||||||||||||||||||||||||

Rich and fluffy pancakes with just the right heat to kick you up to a good start. Man up and give this a shot!

DETAILS:

- Preparation Time: 5 minutes
- Cooking Time: 10 minutes
- Serves: 4

NUTRITIONAL VALUES:

- Kcal per serve: 230
- Fat: 19 g. (76%)
- Protein: 10 g. (20%)
- Carbs: 2 g. (4%)

INGREDIENTS:

- ½ cup Cream Cheese
- 4 Eggs
- ½ cup Almond Flour
- 1 tbsp Minced Jalapenos

PREPARATION:

1. Mix all ingredients in a blender.
2. Preheat a skillet and coat with non-stick spray.
3. Ladle in the batter and cook for 1-2 minutes per side.

. Coconut Chia Pancakes

||||||||||||||||||||||||||||||||||||||||||||||||

et your fat and fiber fix early in the day with a pancake for breakfast that's just as packed in avor as it is in nutrients. This one is highly recommended.

DETAILS:

- Preparation Time: 5 minutes
- Cooking Time: 10 minutes
- Serves: 4

NUTRITIONAL VALUES:

- Kcal per serve: 333
- Fat: 30 g. (79%)
- Protein: 10 g. (14%)
- Carbs: 6 g. (7%)

INGREDIENTS:

- ½ cup Coconut Flour
- 4 Eggs
- 1 cup Coconut Milk
- 1 tsp Psyllium Husk
- ½ tsp Baking Powder
- 1 tbsp Coconut Oil
- 1 tbsp Chia Seeds

PREPARATION:

1. Mix all ingredients in a blender.
2. Preheat a skillet and coat with non-stick spray.
3. Ladle in the batter and cook for 1-2 minutes per side.

4. Keto Blueberry Pancakes

||||||||||||||||||||||||||||||||||||||||||||||||

Get your dose of antioxidants with nothing from the best source nature has given. Yep, those berries are best for your breakfast pancakes too.

DETAILS:

- Preparation Time: 10 minutes
- Cooking Time: 10 minutes
- Serves: 4

NUTRITIONAL VALUES:

- Kcal per serve: 287
- Fat: 25 g. (79%)
- Protein: 11 g. (16%)
- Carbs: 4 g. (5%)

INGREDIENTS:

- ½ cup Cream Cheese
- 4 Eggs
- 2 tbsp Melted Butter
- ½ cup Almond Flour
- 2 tbsp Erythritol
- 1 tsp Baking Powder
- ¼ tsp Salt
- ¼ cup Fresh Blueberries

PREPARATION:

1. Whisk together almond flour, baking powder, and salt in a bowl.
2. In a separate bowl, mix together cream cheese, eggs, butter, and erythritol.
3. Gradually stir in the dry ingredients into the wet mixture.
4. Fold in the blueberries.
5. Preheat a skillet and coat with non-stick spray.
6. Ladle in the batter and cook for 1-2 minutes per side.

5. Spiced Pumpkin Pancakes

Wake up to the soothing aromas as soon as that batter hits the hot pan. You're definitely in for an early morning treat!

DETAILS:

- Preparation Time: 10 minutes
- Cooking Time: 10 minutes
- Serves: 4

NUTRITIONAL VALUES:

- Kcal per serve: 280
- Fat: 23 g. (70%)
- Protein: 12 g. (17%)
- Carbs: 9 g. (13%)

INGREDIENTS:

- 1 cup Almond Flour
- 1 tbsp Pumpkin Pie Spice
- ½ tsp Baking Powder
- 2 tbsp Erythritol
- 3 Eggs
- ¼ cup Pumpkin Puree
- ¼ cup Coconut Milk

PREPARATION:

1. Mix all ingredients in a blender.
2. Preheat a skillet and coat with non-stick spray.
3. Ladle in the batter and cook for 1-2 minutes per side.

6. Low-Carb Red Velvet Pancakes

||||||||||||||||||||||||||||||||||||||||||||||||||

Red velvet inspired pancakes that's guaranteed low in carbs. Yes of course, the goodness of cacao and cream cheese are in here too.

DETAILS:

- Preparation Time: 5 minutes
- Cooking Time: 10 minutes
- Serves: 4

NUTRITIONAL VALUES:

- Kcal per serve: 339
- Fat: 29 g. (77%)
- Protein: 13 g. (17%)
- Carbs: 5 g. (6%)

INGREDIENTS:

- ½ cup Cream Cheese
- 4 Eggs
- 2 tbsp Butter, melted
- ½ cup Almond Flour
- 1 tbsp Unsweetened Cocoa Powder
- 2 tbsp Erythritol
- 1 tsp Vanilla Extract
- ½ tsp Red Food Coloring

PREPARATION:

1. Mix all ingredients in a blender.
2. Preheat a skillet and coat with non-stick spray.
3. Ladle in the batter and cook for 1-2 minutes per side.

. Citrus and Ricotta Pancakes

||||||||||||||||||||||||||||||||||||||||||||||||||

ight and delicate ricotta-enriched pancakes with a bright touch of citrus flavor. Mornings are
st meant to be bright, right?

ETAILS:

- Preparation Time: 5 minutes
- Cooking Time: 10 minutes
- Serves: 4

NUTRITIONAL VALUES:

- Kcal per serve: 256
- Fat: 20 g. (68%)
- Protein: 15 g. (25%)
- Carbs: 5 g. (7%)

NGREDIENTS:

- ½ cup Ricotta Cheese
- 4 Eggs
- ½ cup Almond Flour
- 1 tsp Orange Zest
- 1 tsp Vanilla Extract

PREPARATION:

1. Mix all ingredients in a blender.
2. Preheat a skillet and coat with non-stick spray.
3. Ladle in the batter and cook for 1-2 minutes per side.

8. Keto Bacon and Cheese Pancakes

||||||||||||||||||||||||||||||||||||||||||||||||||

With bacon and cheddar in a pancake, could there just be a more perfect breakfast than this? Not so much, and that's for sure.

DETAILS:

- Preparation Time: 10 minutes
- Cooking Time: 10 minutes
- Serves: 4

NUTRITIONAL VALUES:

- Kcal per serve: 290
- Fat: 22 g. (67%)
- Protein: 17 g. (24%)
- Carbs: 6 g. (8%)

INGREDIENTS:

- ½ cup Shredded Cheddar
- 4 Eggs, separated
- ½ cup Almond Flour
- ½ tsp Cream of Tartar
- ¼ tsp Salt
- ¼ cup Bacon Bits
- 1 tbsp Chopped Chives

PREPARATION:

1. Whisk the egg whites and cream of tartar until soft peaks from.
2. Sift in the almond flour and salt.
3. Fold in the cheddar, bacon, and chives.
4. Lightly coat a non-stick pan with cooking spray.
5. Ladle the batter in and cook for 1-2 minutes per side.

. Keto Avocado Pancakes

|||||||||||||||||||||||||||||||||||||||||||||||||||

ll the keto-favored fat of ripe avocados whisked up in a pancake batter. Simply excellent.

DETAILS:

- Preparation Time: 5 minutes
- Cooking Time: 10 minutes
- Serves: 4

NUTRITIONAL VALUES:

- Kcal per serve: 199
- Fat: 16 g. (70%)
- Protein: 7 g. (16%)
- Carbs: 7 g. (14%)

INGREDIENTS:

- 1 Large Avocado
- 2 Eggs
- ½ cup Milk
- ¼ cup Almond Flour
- ½ tsp Baking Powder
- 1 tbsp Erythritol

PREPARATION:

1. Mix all ingredients in a blender.
2. Preheat a skillet and coat with non-stick spray.
3. Ladle in the batter and cook for 1-2 minutes per side.

10. Purple Yam Pancakes

||||||||||||||||||||||||||||||||||||||||||||||||

Purple pancakes anyone? And it ain't all about the inviting color. Those yams give these pancakes a depth of flavor like no other.

DETAILS:

- Preparation Time: 5 minutes
- Cooking Time: 10 minutes
- Serves: 4

NUTRITIONAL VALUES:

- Kcal per serve: 347
- Fat: 31 g. (76%)
- Protein: 11 g. (13%)
- Carbs: 9 g. (11%)

INGREDIENTS:

- ½ cup Coconut Flour
- 4 Eggs
- 1 cup Coconut Milk
- 1 tsp Guar Gum
- ½ tsp Baking Powder
- 1 tbsp Coconut Oil
- ¼ cup Purple Yam Puree

PREPARATION:

1. Mix all ingredients in a blender.
2. Preheat a skillet and coat with non-stick spray.
3. Ladle in the batter and cook for 1-2 minutes per side.

No-Bake

1. No-Bake Carrot Cake

||||||||||||||||||||||||||||||||||||||||||||||||||||

Yup, the so popular carrot cake can be had in a no-bake , no-fuss, ketogenic version too! If you're a fan of this traditional treat then look no further.

DETAILS:

- Preparation Time: 1 hour
- Cooking Time:
- Serves: 6

NUTRITIONAL VALUES:

- Kcal per serve: 257
- Fat: 23 g. (80%)
- Protein: 5 g. (8%)
- Carbs: 8 g. (12%)

INGREDIENTS:

- 150 grams Carrots, finely grated
- 1 cup Cream Cheese, softened
- ½ cup Ground Almonds
- ½ cup Ground Walnuts
- ½ cup Shredded Coconut
- 1 tsp Cinnamon Powder
- ¼ tsp Nutmeg
- ¼ tsp Ground Cardamom

PREPARATION:

1. Combine all ingredients in a bowl. Mix until well combined.
2. Press the mixture into cupcake molds and freeze for an hour to set.

. No-Bake Keto Brownies

||||||||||||||||||||||||||||||||||||||||||||||||||

quick and easy chocolate fix for all you cocoa junkies out there. And this recipe would serve e weight watchers too given the insignificant amount of net carbs in every serving of these rownies.

DETAILS:

- Preparation Time: 1 hour
- Cooking Time:
- Serves: 12

NUTRITIONAL VALUES:

- Kcal per serve: 109
- Fat: 12 g. (97%)
- Protein: 1 g. (1%)
- Carbs: 1 g. (2%)

INGREDIENTS:

- 1 cup Almond Flour
- ¼ cup Unsweetened Cocoa Powder
- ¾ cup Erythritol
- ¾ cup Butter, softened
- 1 tbsp Vanilla extract

PREPARATION:

1. Combine all ingredients in a bowl. Mix until well combined.
2. Press the mixture into a rectangular silicon mold and freeze for an hour to set.
3. Slice for serving.

3. No-Bake Keto Cheesecake

||||||||||||||||||||||||||||||||||||||||||||||||||||

Just as rich and delicate as any cheesecake you could ask for. This is simply heaven for those on a keto diet.

DETAILS:

- Preparation Time: 1 hour
- Cooking Time:
- Serves: 8

NUTRITIONAL VALUES:

- Kcal per serve: 459
- Fat: 45 g. (86%)
- Protein: 10 g. (8%)
- Carbs: 8 g. (6%)

INGREDIENTS:

For the Crust

- 2 cups Almond Flour
- ¼ cup Erythritol
- 1 tsp Cinnamon Powder
- ½ cup Coconut Oil

For the Filling

- 2 cups Cream Cheese
- ½ cup Erythritol
- 1 tsp Vanilla Extract
- 1 tsp Lemon Zest
- 1 tbsp Gelatin
- 1 cup Boiling Water

PREPARATION:

1. Combine all ingredients for the crust in a bowl. Mix well. Pack the mixture into a 9-inch springform pan.
2. Combine gelatin and erythritol in a bowl. Stir in a cup of boiling water. Leave for 5 minutes.
3. Beat cream cheese and vanilla in a separate bowl until light and airy.
4. Gradually stir in the gelatin mixture into the whipped cream cheese. Fold in the lemon zest.
5. Chill the mixture for 30 minutes then spread onto the crust.
6. Set the prepared cake in the chiller until ready to serve.

1. No-Bake Peanut Butter Cookies

|||||||||||||||||||||||||||||||||||||||||||||||||||||||

ust mix, shape, and chill. I'm sure we all sneaked into that raw cookie dough in the kitchen as 'ds.

DETAILS:

- Preparation Time: 1 hour
- Cooking Time:
- Serves: 6

NUTRITIONAL VALUES:

- Kcal per serve: 289
- Fat: 21 g. (65%)
- Protein: 19 g. (26%)
- Carbs: 6 g. (9%)

INGREDIENTS:

- 1 cup Peanut Butter
- 2 tbsp Almond Flour
- 1 tbsp Erythritol
- 1/3 cup Sugar-Free Chocolate Chips

PREPARATION:

1. Combine all ingredients in a bowl. Mix until well combined.
2. Scoop the dough into balls and flatten slightly onto a tray lined with parchment.
3. Freeze for 30 minutes to set.

5. No-Bake Coconut Bars

||||||||||||||||||||||||||||||||||||||||||||||||||||||

Packed with all the healthy fats from coconuts and of course that unique nutty taste. These yummy bars surely won't disappoint.

DETAILS:

- Preparation Time: 1 hour
- Cooking Time:
- Serves: 5

NUTRITIONAL VALUES:

- Kcal per serve: 136
- Fat: 13 g. (84%)
- Protein: 1 g. (4%)
- Carbs: 4 g. (12%)

INGREDIENTS:

- 1 cup Shredded Coconut
- ½ cup Coconut Cream
- ½ cup Erythritol

PREPARATION:

1. Combine all ingredients in a bowl. Mix until well combined.
2. Press the mixture into a rectangular silicon mold and freeze for an hour to set.
3. Slice for serving.

. No-Bake Keto Mousse Cake

||||||||||||||||||||||||||||||||||||||||||||||

eep chocolate flavor with every smooth and delicate bite. This low-carb mousse is to die for.

DETAILS:

- Preparation Time: 1 hour
- Cooking Time:
- Serves: 8

NUTRITIONAL VALUES:

- Kcal per serve: 400
- Fat: 38 g. (84%)
- Protein: 8 g. (7%)
- Carbs: 10 g. (9%)

INGREDIENTS:

For the Crust

- 1.5 cups Almond Flour
- ¼ cup Unsweetened Cocoa Powder
- ¼ cup Erythritol
- ½ cup Melted Butter

For the Filling

- 1.5 cups Cream Cheese
- ½ cup Dark Chocolate Chips, melted
- ½ cup Erythritol
- 1 tsp Vanilla Extract
- 1 tbsp Gelatin
- 1 cup Boiling Water

PREPARATION:

1. Combine all ingredients for the crust in a bowl. Mix well. Pack the mixture into a 9-inch springform pan.
2. Combine gelatin and erythritol in a bowl. Stir in a cup of boiling water. Leave for 5 minutes.
3. Beat cream cheese, melted chocolate, and vanilla in a separate bowl until light and airy.
4. Gradually stir in the gelatin mixture into the cream cheese mixture. Chill the mixture for 30 minutes then spread onto the crust.
5. Set the prepared cake in the chiller until ready to serve.

7. No-Bake Pumpkin Pie

||||||||||||||||||||||||||||||||||||||||||||||||||

*A smooth, nutty, and perfectly spiced pumpkin pie that does not require any baking skills. Ev[en]
the kids can do this!*

DETAILS:

- Preparation Time: 8 hours
- Cooking Time:
- Serves: 8

NUTRITIONAL VALUES:

- Kcal per serve: 315
- Fat: 29 g. (80%)
- Protein: 7 g. (8%)
- Carbs: 9 g. (12%)

INGREDIENTS:

For the Crust

- 1 cup Walnuts, chopped
- 1 cup Almond Flour
- ¼ cup Erythritol
- 1/3 cup Melted Butter

For the Filling

- 1 14-oz can Pumpkin Puree
- ½ cup Erythritol
- 1 cup Heavy Cream
- 6 Egg Yolks
- 1 tbsp Gelatin
- 1 tsp Vanilla Extract
- 1 tsp Cinnamon Powder
- ¼ tsp Ground Ginger
- ¼ tsp Ground Nutmeg
- ¼ tsp Ground Cloves

PREPARATION:

1. Combine all ingredients for the crust in a bowl. Mix well. Pack the mixture into a 9-inch springform pan.
2. Combine all ingredients for the filling in a pot. Whisk over medium heat until mixture starts to thicken.
3. Pour filling into the crust and refrigerate overnight.

6. No-Bake Tiramisu Cups

||||||||||||||||||||||||||||||||||||||||||||||||||||

the French thought putting together espresso and mascarpone in a single treat was genius, en making the very same dessert low-carb is even more clever. Enjoy. . .free of guilt.

DETAILS:

- Preparation Time: 2 hours
- Cooking Time:
- Serves: 8

NUTRITIONAL VALUES:

- Kcal per serve: 364
- Fat: 37 g. (89%)
- Protein: 5 g. (5%)
- Carbs: 5 g. (5%)

INGREDIENTS:

For the Crust

- 1 cup Pecans, ground
- 1/3 cup Melted Butter
- 1 tbsp Unsweetened Cocoa Powder
- 2 tbsp Erythritol

For the Filling

- 2 cups Mascarpone Cheese
- 1 shot Espresso
- ½ cup Erythritol
- 1 tsp Vanilla Extract
- 1 tbsp Gelatin
- 1 cup Boiling Water

PREPARATION:

1. Combine all ingredients for the crust in a bowl. Mix well. Pack the mixture into a silicon cupcake mold.
2. Combine gelatin and erythritol in a bowl. Stir in a cup of boiling water. Leave for 5 minutes.
3. Beat mascarpone cheese, espresso, and vanilla in a separate bowl until light and airy.
4. Gradually stir in the gelatin mixture into the whipped mascarpone.
5. Chill the mixture for 30 minutes.
6. Divide the mixture onto the cupcake mold and chill for an hour.

9. No-Bake Choco-Chip Blondies

||||||||||||||||||||||||||||||||||||||||||||||||||||||

Unbelievably low in carbs for something dense and delicious. Skip counting those macros, these no-bake blondies are truly keto-friendly.

DETAILS:

- Preparation Time: 1 hour
- Cooking Time:
- Serves: 12

NUTRITIONAL VALUES:

- Kcal per serve: 170
- Fat: 14 g. (73%)
- Protein: 5 g. (11%)
- Carbs: 7 g. (16%)

INGREDIENTS:

- 1 cup Almond Flour
- ¾ cup Erythritol
- ¾ cup Almond Butter
- 1 tbsp Vanilla extract
- ½ cup Sugar-Free Chocolate Chips

PREPARATION:

1. Mix together almond butter, coconut flour, erythritol, and vanilla extract in a bowl until well combined.
2. Fold in the chocolate chips.
3. Press the mixture into a rectangular silicon mold and freeze for an hour to set.
4. Slice for serving.

0. No-Bake Banana Bread

||||||||||||||||||||||||||||||||||||||||||||||||||

Always craved for a sweet and fragrant slice of banana bread but too worried about all the sugar? This might just be the recipe you've been looking for.

DETAILS:

- Preparation Time: 1 hour
- Cooking Time:
- Serves: 8

NUTRITIONAL VALUES:

- Kcal per serve: 116
- Fat: 8 g. (61%)
- Protein: 2 g. (8%)
- Carbs: 9 g. (31%)

INGREDIENTS:

- 2 Medium Bananas, mashed
- ½ cup Coconut Flour
- ¼ cup Almond Butter
- 2 tbsp Erythritol
- ¼ cup Chopped Walnuts

PREPARATION:

1. Combine all ingredients in a bowl. Mix until well combined.
2. Press the mixture into cupcake molds and freeze for an hour to set.

Conclusion

There you have it, a complete collection of low carb, Keto friendly, gluten-free breads that you can make and serve for a variety of meals or occasions. As you saw, each of the recipes in this book is incredibly easy to follow, and most of them are also incredibly inexpensive to make.

These breads are made using the normal ingredients you can find locally, so there's no need to have to order anything, or have to go to any specialty stores for any of them. With these breads you can enjoy the same meals you used to enjoy, but stay on track with your diet as much as yo want.

Lose the weight you want to lose, feel great, and still get to indulge in that piping hot piece of bread every now and then. Spread on your favorite topping, and your bread craving will be satisfied.

I hope the recipes in this book were able to inspire you to take your own baking to the next level As you can see by each of these, you can alter and modify a variety of things to give them that custom spin you need from time to time.

Are you ready to enjoy those breads as you once did? Are you ready to serve soup or salad with a side of breadsticks or rolls? Are you ready to have a pizza night once again?

You know you are, so what are you waiting for? Grab your apron and preheat your oven. Get your ingredients and the mixing bowl, and you're set to have your bread and eat it, too!

Free Bonus

Thank you for purchasing this cookbook! As a token of my appreciation, I want to give one of my favorite cookbooks for free – "Keto Smoothies: Delicious High-Fat Smoothies To Lose Weight, Boost Energy and Brain Power"

It shows you how to make delicious keto smoothies without ever going out of ketosis. I make these smoothies every day!

To download it, go to HTTPS://WWW.NJKETO.COM/SMOOTHIES and sign up.

After signing up download link will be delivered straight to your mailbox.

By signing up you also agree to receive occasional goodness packed emails from me.

Thank you for reading and enjoying my keto cookbooks!

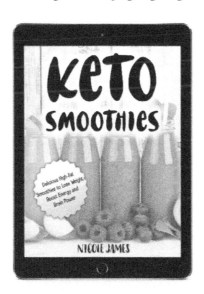

VISIT

HTTPS://WWW.NJKETO.COM/SMOOTHIES

FOR A FREE DOWNLOAD!

Made in the USA
Las Vegas, NV
25 November 2022